REFLECTIONS DURING THE COVID-19 PANDEMIC

URBANISM BEYOND 2020

Vinayak Bharne

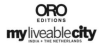

Contents

01
___

Our Health and the City

02
___

The Forest and the City

03
___

The Wild City

04
___

The Unfair City

05
___

The Informal City

06
___

The Privilege of Community

07
___

Governance Matters

08
___

Paradigms of Open Space

For my father, **Mohanlal Bharne**,
who among other things, taught me
to communicate and write

Introduction

This book contains excerpts from talks I gave during the COVID-19 lockdowns. Between January 2020 and June 2021, as we all grappled with the pandemic, I received more invites to participate (via digital media) in architecture and urbanism forums than before. In the process of preparing for them, I realized that my notes, though instigated by the pandemic, were in fact seeking to emphasize numerous issues I consider crucial to city making today - compelling me to write them more systematically as short essays.

The pandemic has highlighted many fundamental aspects about our built environment. It has reminded us why city making is a health project. It has affirmed the inextricable relationship between ecological and human wellbeing. It has underscored the insurmountable damage we have inflicted on our natural environment and shown us that we consume a lot more than we actually need. It has revealed how unjust and unfair our cities are, how a sudden crisis affects us all differently, and how leadership, governance, and administration play a crucial role in our reception of difficult circumstances.

Simultaneously, the pandemic has helped demonstrate how resilient, adaptable, and ingenious our cities can be during uncertain times. It has helped renew our relationship with our dwellings, buildings, and neighborhoods. It has instigated serious rethinking on our urban habituations and their impact on the natural environment, and inspired ideas about how we might transform them toward greater collective goals. It has shown us that we live in an interconnected, interdependent world.

Urbanism Beyond 2020 is an attempt to reflect on what living with this pandemic has suggested about our urban future. Amidst climate change, widening socio-economic gaps, and this crisis on the one hand, and increasing cross-cultural and economic fluidity on the other, the myriad issues shaping cities across the world today, and the numerous ways in which cities are coming to terms with them have a lot to teach us all. Cities with limited means offer incredible lessons on resilience and resourcefulness to affluent societies that take their prosperity for granted. In turn, the virtues of effective urban administration, regulation, and accountability seen in developed societies can reassuringly serve to inspire less developed ones. The pointers to our future will not emerge exclusively from affluent nations, or less developed societies alone.

To this end, the 20 essays in this book traverse places and examples that are geographically, culturally, and economically diverse. They go from India, where I was born, to the United States, where I currently reside, to Brazil, China, Colombia, Japan, Nepal, Spain, the Philippines, the Netherlands, New Zealand, and Uganda, where I have taught, designed projects, or conducted research.

The essays touch upon a variety of topics - ecology, wildlife, social justice, vernacular habitats, the water crisis, public space, urban density, informal economies, governance, religion, and urban art - because you cannot look at something as complex as cities from a singular perspective. As a practicing urban designer and city planner trained in architecture, this plural and global outlook has been an invaluable litmus test and feedback loop. Just as you think you know something about cities, you discover an aspect that contradicts it.

The term "Urbanism" in this book is meant to describe the science and art of making cities, as both product and process. On the one hand, cities are shaped by physical elements such as public spaces, buildings, and infrastructural systems - largely the canvas of architects, landscape architects, urban designers, and engineers. On the other hand, cities are shaped through non-physical means such a policy, activism, advocacy, and administration - the domain of politicians, civic leaders, urban planners, and citizen-groups. The term therefore refers to a mesh of entities, disciplines, and aspects that generate our cities.

The content of this volume springs from many global events that occurred during the lockdowns. To begin with, the book's cover depicts my rendition of a city gradually coalescing to normalcy after being shaken up by the pandemic. Will our cities emerge from this shocking crisis wiser and more empathetic? Then, to set the stage for a reader, there is a chart before the book's Introduction titled "2020 at a Glance" - a sweeping reminder of the first twelve months during which our desperate world struggled and came to grips with the pandemic in different ways.

The twenty essays that follow do not appear in the sequence in which they were delivered as lectures. I have intentionally left them undated, because I feel they are broad enough to withstand the test of time. Though some of them touch upon specific events that were occurring during the lockdowns, I felt that organizing the essays according to their themes would make for a more compelling narrative. I begin with an essay titled "Our Health and the City"- a rather obvious starting point. I conclude with "The Pawn and the Chess Game," reflecting on architectural and urbanist practice in the hopes that this collection will inspire not just further thought, but action towards positive change.

In my list of acknowledgements, I would like to begin with Shyam Khandekar and Shashikala Venkatraman, co-founders of the

India-Netherlands-based knowledge-platform, My Liveable City. Shyam read my earliest essays, encouraged me to collect them into a book, and along with Shashi, supported the idea of this publication. Gordon Goff and Jake Anderson of ORO Editions accommodated my delays with great patience. And my former student, Apurva Ravi, enthusiastically designed this volume and its graphics from cover to cover.

My thoughts in this book have evolved over the years from talks and articles that were the result of invitations from numerous organizations. As an act of gratitude for giving me a platform, I would like to mention some of them: In India - Sunapranta: Goa Center for the Arts; The Marg Foundation; School of Planning & Architecture (New Delhi, Bhopal, Vijaywada); CEPT University; Banaras Hindu University; Indian Institute of Architects; Institute of Town Planners India; and the Indian Society of Landscape Architects. In China - South China Agricultural University; and China Architectural Heritage. In Japan - Kyoto Journal; and Japan Foundation. In Europe - Institute for Housing and Urban Development Studies, Erasmus University (The Netherlands); Journal of Architecture and Urbanism (UK); The Urban Design Group (UK); and University of Ljubljana (Slovenia). In the United States - Association of Collegiate Schools of Architecture; Journal of Architectural Education; DOCOMOMO; Parsons School of Design; University of Wisconsin Milwaukee; University of California Los Angeles; University of Southern California; University of Illinois Chicago; American Planning Association; and Congress for the New Urbanism. In Africa - U for Urban Impact (Egypt). And in Australia - The Australian Urban Forum.

Over the years, various individuals have been invaluable discussants on urbanism: Aseem Inam (professor of Urban Design, Cardiff University); Shyam Khandekar (co-founder of My Liveable City); Rana P. B. Singh (former professor of geography, Banaras Hindu University); Nihal Perera (professor of Urban Planning, Ball State University); Trudi Sandmeier (director of the Heritage Conservation program, University of Southern California); Poonam Verma Mascarenhas (director, Archinova-Environs); John Torti (president, Torti Gallas & Partners); John Dutton (principal, Dutton Architects); Alan Loomis (principal, Placeworks); Yo Hakomori (principal, StudioHAU); and Dhiru Thadani (principal, Thadani Architects & Urbanists).

I wish to acknowledge four mentors who have in different ways shaped my understanding of cities and urbanism: 1) Bruno Dias Souza - a student of Josep Lluis Sert at Harvard University in the 1950s - who inspired me to be globally curious during my under-graduate years in India; 2) Robert (Bob) Harris, my teacher at, and former dean of, the University of Southern California (USC) School of Architecture, who solidified my understanding of the interrela-tionship between architecture and the city; 3) Tridib Banerjee - a protégé of Kevin Lynch at the Massachusetts Institute of Tech-nology and former professor at the USC Price School of Public Policy - who nudged me to explore less studied cities; and 4) Stefanos Polyzoides - co-founder of the Congress for the New Urbanism - with whom I have journeyed on many adventures in professional practice. Whether or not I fully subscribe to their thoughts, I will always carry a little bit of them with me.

On a personal note, this book would not have been possible without the love and support of my wife Paige, and my children Sebastian and Portia. My in-laws Nancy and Peter Kemball tuned in to listen to many of my talks and read some of the essays, and I remain grateful for their affection and support.

Finally, I express gratitude to my parents. My mother, Neela Bharne, taught me about the importance of compassion and empathy. My father, Mohanlal Bharne, taught me to communicate and write. He passed away in April 2021 during the making of this book. I dedicate this book to him.

Vinayak Bharne
Los Angeles, July 2021

2020 at a Glance

January

(9) World Health Organization announces coronavirus-related pneumonia in the city of Wuhan, China

(23) The cities of Wuhan and Huanggang with a total of 18 million people are under quarantine

(30) The World Health Organization declares COVID-19 a Public Health Emergency of International Concern at a meeting in Geneva

February

(2) Air travel restrictions imposed by the United States, Australia, Germany, Italy and New Zealand

(3) A 1000-bed COVID-19 hospital built in just 10 days opens its doors in Wuhan, China

(14) First confirmed COVID-19 case on the African continent in Egypt

May

(13) Every country on the African continent is reported to have cases of COVID-19

(19) A study published in Nature Climate Change reports a 17% drop in greenhouse emissions worldwide during the lockdowns

(28) The Boston Marathon is cancelled for the first time in its 123-year history

June

(4) Brazil surpasses Italy with the third-highest COVID-19 death toll

(8) New Zealand reports no active cases, with the last remaining patient reported to have recovered

(20) Highest ever temperature of 38 degrees centigrade (100 degrees fahrenheit) recorded in Verkhoyansk, Siberia

September

(2) Australia officially declares recession for the first time in almost 3 decades

(14) Israel becomes the first country to announce a second national lockdown due to COVID-19

(28) Global COVID-19 deaths surpass 1 million

October

(9) The United Nation's World Food Program is awarded the Nobel Peace Prize

(17) Jacinda Ardern is re-elected as New Zealand's prime minister in a landslide election

(26) Pakistan's first metro line, the Orange Line, opens in the city of Lahore

March

(11) World Health Organization declares COVID-19 a pandemic

(23) The government of India orders a nationwide 21-day lockdown, limiting the movement of 1.3 billion people

(27) Panamanian authorities stop a Dutch-American cruise ship, the MS Zandam, with two confirmed COVID-19 cases, from entering the Panama Canal

April

(2) Number of COVID-19 cases worldwide passes 1 million

(14) The Indian government extends India's COVID-19 lockdown until May 3

(17) Art galleries reopen along the Bund in Shanghai, China, for the first time since the lockdown

July

(17) The Gion Matsuri, one of Japan's biggest festivals held annually in Kyoto is cancelled

(24) India reports a new record-high 49,000-plus COVID-19 cases in 24 hours

(31) The Apple wildfire starts near Beaumont, California, forcing the evacuation of nearly 8000 people

August

(6) COVID-19 detected cases in Africa pass 1 million

(29) The Metropolitan Museum of Art in New York reopens

(30) Global coronavirus cases top 25-million

November

(7) Joseph R. Biden is elected 46th president of the United States of America

(16) United States pharmaceutical company Moderna says its COVID-19 vaccine is 94.5% effective

(28) Thousands of farmers gather in Delhi, India, to protest proposed agriculture reforms

December

(7) The International Olympic Committee deeds to make competitive breakdancing an Olympic sport.

(8) A grandmother in the United Kingdom becomes the world's first person to be given a COVID-19 vaccine

(31) Per Worldometer.info, the total number of COVID-19 related deaths worldwide is 1,834,795

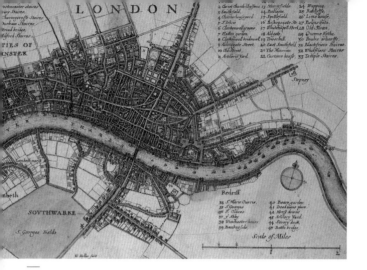

Figure 1.1

Plan of London before the September 1666 Great Fire, by Wenceslaus Hollar (1607-1677). Source: Public Domain

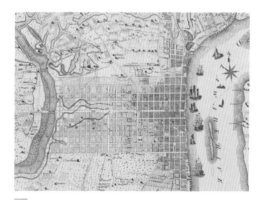

Figure 1.2

Plan of Philadelphia, circa 1796, from Charles D. Kaufmann's 1895 Street Atlas of Philadelphia by wards. Source: Public Domain

01

Our Health and the City

The COVID-19 pandemic has brought human fragility and mortality to our psychological forefront. By the time the first vaccine was delivered to an individual in early December 2020, the pandemic had taken the lives of more than 1.6 million people across the world within a single year. As such, the pandemic has highlighted the most fundamental aspect of our existence - our health. It has redirected our attention to the relationship between our collective and individual well-being and the built environments in which we live.

We are not strangers to epidemics and pandemics. The Black Death killed millions in the 14th century. Increasing transportation in the late 1800s spread influenza across the globe. The Swine Flu killed more than 500,000 people in 2009. From 2015–2016, the Zika virus spread from Brazil to parts of South and North America and Southeast Asia. Epidemics and pandemics have ravaged humanity before. But they have also offered profound insights on the connections between our habitats and what we call disease, and instigated strategies to enable us to endure health crises.

For example, William Penn, the founder of Philadelphia, one of the first great planned cities in the United States, had survived the plague and Great Fire of London in the 1660s. Concerned that tenuous non-rectilinear street patterns were susceptible to stagnating water, he planned the new city in 1682 as a rectangular grid of streets headed toward the Delaware River. Each house was placed in the middle of a large lot surrounded by open space on all sides, and each quadrant featured a public square to prevent overcrowding and allow ample sunlight and cross ventilation.

The cholera outbreak in London instigated the 1848 Public Health Act with the establishment of the general Board of Health. Subsequently, social reformer Edwin Chadwick who became an officer of the London Metropolitan Sewers Commission ordered all cesspools and sewage pits to be cleared from the streets and dumped into the Thames - whose inevitable result was the Great Stink of 1858. This in turn led to Joseph Bazalgette's 1877 engineering solution of channeling the waste through miles of street sewers into intercepting sewers so that it could be transported downstream into the tidal water of the Thames River and swept out to sea.

When yellow fever infected its residents in 1878, the city of Memphis, Tennessee, undertook a detailed citywide lot-by-lot survey prepared by a diverse team of experts. Engineers inspected buildings for new code requirements. Doctors helped identify places that could be susceptible to disease, and planners sought strategies to decongest over-crowded neighborhoods by designing parks and green spaces. The epidemic had forced the city to recognize the need for a significant public health strategy through multi-disciplinary collaboration to prevent another health crisis.

In the mid to late 1800s, increasing density and population in the early industrial city instilled fear of catching disease via foul air, and buildings and outdoor areas with fresh air and sunlight became a priority. For example, Manhattan's grid was originally designed in 1811 without parks and it was not until the late 1840s, when the North American city was growing due to industrialization and immigration, that leaders began to call for green space. The result was the nation's first great urban park, Central Park, conceived by

Frederick Law Olmsted and built in 1858 as the "Lungs of the City." The creation of parklands was so intimately intertwined with public health that Olmsted left his post as superintendent of Central Park to become general secretary of the United States Sanitary Commission - which would become the nation's largest national public health effort.

With increasing industrialization, the physical separation of noxious uses like slaughterhouses and steel plants from places where people resided, overlapped with important medical discoveries that had a direct impact on city making. For instance, in 1897, British doctor Ronald Ross's discovery of the malaria parasite in the gastrointestinal tract of a mosquito had a significant impact on urban design and planning. In colonial India, circa 1931, the city of New Delhi was built to be physically disconnected from the older labyrinthine 17th-century walled city of Shahajahanabad. A hygienic zone in the form of a vast open space separated the two, and its width was carefully calculated per the maximum flight distance of the malaria-spreading Anopheles mosquito.

Meanwhile, sanitarians had started filling up urban tanks and village reservoirs in colonial India to prevent mosquito breeding, a trend that was criticized by British town planner Patrick Geddes. The cooling effect that the reservoirs had on their habitat surroundings, and the cultural significance of these water bodies to the indigenous demographic had not escaped him. He argued for more ecologically sensitive approaches such as "clean(ing) them thoroughly and then stock(ing) them with sufficient fish and duck to keep down the Anopheles" while noting that the "cleansing of tanks costs but a fraction of the cost of filling them." Geddes's wisdom, stemming in part from his training as a biologist, was far ahead of its times. He was reinforcing how the fields of city planning and public health were intertwined with other environmental, social, and technical sciences, all working hand-in-hand toward a holistic vision for a healthy city.

But with the over-bureaucratization of municipal governments and the increased specialization of engineering fields, multiple disciplines with broader overlapping goals became increasingly less-communicative - and the COVID-19 pandemic has exposed this gap. Today, our urban development patterns are detrimental to our health. Urban policies and zoning codes, over recent decades, have enabled entire communities that have no access to healthy food, and that rely on the car, discouraging people to walk, and leading to increasing obesity, asthma, and heart disease. Homes, schools, and even day-care centers are built adjacent to toxic free-ways contributing to the growing list of our health problems. The global syndrome of overburdened hospitals, lack of infrastructural upgrade, increasing pressure on healthcare professionals, and the absence of healthcare for the underprivileged is also an extension of this discipline separation. And even in the most developed soci-eties of the world, this occurs legally, through policy and regulation.

Like before, the pandemic is instigating serious questions on our cities from a health perspective: Will social distancing generate a more polycentric urban landscape with daily needs within walking distance of our homes? Will it incentivize the creation of more public open spaces? Will it encourage our dwellings to be naturally ventilated, and discourage air-tight buildings? Simultaneously, the pandemic is raising concerns: Will returning to the inner city - an increasing trend over the past two decades - wane as people seek more pastoral places to reside? How will the informal sector and its unplanned habitats cope with this crisis? Numerous questions in kind are already part of significant dialogues as we come to terms with what this pandemic means for our future.

As we contemplate such questions, we must not fail to notice the pandemic's numerous silver linings. During the lockdowns, we have been forced to rely less on our cars. People living in closed build-ings are spending more time outdoors. Awareness of personal and public hygiene has seen a surge, particularly with health authorities advocating for regular handwashing, and there is a good chance this will not wear off easily. In the post-COVID-19 city we will expect our municipal leaders and health departments to be better prepared and far more invested in disease preparedness and response. And so, it may be that our digital interactions for business and work, renewed sense of personal and communal health, and calculated frugality in daily habits are not only an effective but also an environmentally-friendly way to live after this global pandemic has passed.

Inasmuch as this pandemic has startled us all, it has also made us realize that our pre-COVID-19 urban patterns were neither good for our health, nor that of our planet - and the two are inextricably interrelated. After a long time, the air we breathe in our cities is cleaner, our forests and oceans are less disturbed than they have been in decades, and we are conscious and attentive to what this means for our health. We are beginning to realize that our cities are not just engines for commerce and social life. They are also the conduits and settings for our collective and individual wellness.

The term "wellness" is important here. While health may refer to the absence of disease, it does not always encompass emotional well-being. It does not necessarily include the accumulating toxins in one's body due to an unhealthy diet or lifestyle that have long-term consequences. "Health" is not the end goal but only the first step toward wellness - which is about taking one's health to the highest potential by changing daily habits and being accountable for them.

The means through which our built environments are made and sustained is an intrinsic part of this aspiration, and we must therefore recast them towards achieving these goals. The most significant shift we can hope for in the (post-)COVID-19 world is to return city planning, urban design, and architecture beyond their aesthetic and technical dimensions to their higher and more consequential purpose - as a *health-project* aimed at rejuvenating both human and environmental wellness at all scales.

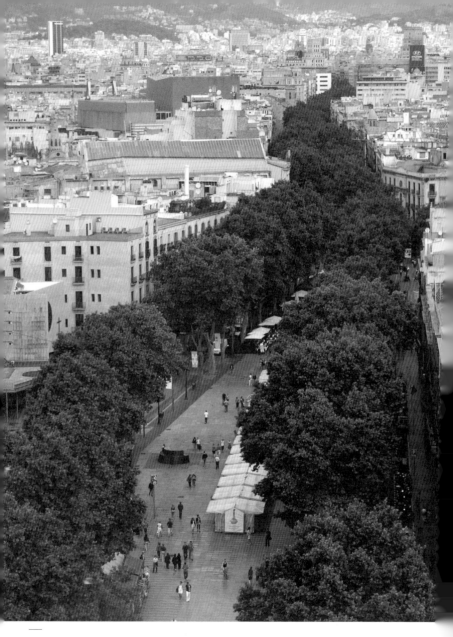

Figure 2.1 **Aerial view of the 1.2 kilometer-long pedestrian street, La Rambla, in Barcelona, Spain.** Source: Nikos Roussos (see Image Credits for details)

The Forest and the City

The human activity lull during the COVID-19 pandemic lockdowns is a period of replenishment, restoration and healing for nature. The onslaught that we continue to inflict on our planet's natural resources is unthinkable. Per the Ocean Conservancy, eight million metric tons of plastic are dumped into our oceans each year, and this is on top of the estimated 150 million metric tons that currently circulate in our marine environments. We have caused the greatest rate of species extinction in the last 65-million years. And our oceans are acidifying faster than they have in more than 300 million years.

Forests still cover about 30 percent of our planet's land area, but they are disappearing at an alarming rate. Per the World Wildlife Fund (WWF), the tropics lost close to 30 soccer fields' worth of trees every single minute in 2019. And according to the World Bank, we have lost 1.3 million square kilometers of forest (larger than the area of South Africa) between 1990 and 2016. In light of this pandemic, herein lies a cause for serious concern - because studies suggest that forest loss is related to the spread of disease from animals to humans.

Recent analysis published in the flagship journal Landscape Ecology by Laura S. P. Bloomfield, Tyler L. McIntosh & Eric F. Lambin has analyzed how forest depletion can increase

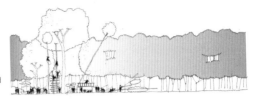

Forest section cleared around selected tree

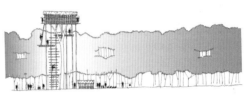

House construction begins and is completed in a few weeks

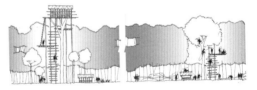

The occupied house is rebuilt in the same location every three to five years until the site no longer allows it

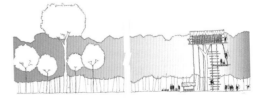

Construction of a new house begins in another part of the forest

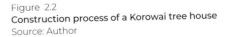

New tree house is occupied. The old house site has rejuvenated itself as forest

Figure 2.2
Construction process of a Korowai tree house
Source: Author

the risk of physical interactions between humans, wild primates, and the viruses they carry. The creation of agricultural land brings settlements to the edge of forested habitats. Humans venture into forests to hunt or collect wood and due to the diminishing forest footprint, animals venture out of their natural habitats in search of food. The source of HIV, for instance, has been identified as a type of chimpanzee in West Africa. The animal's infected blood came into contact with humans who hunted them for meat. The animal's version of the immunodeficiency virus (called simian immunodeficiency virus, or SIV) was most likely transmitted to humans and mutated into HIV.

There is now increasing evidence that the Ebola epidemic that killed thousands across West Africa from 2014–16 was linked to deforestation. It originated in Meliandou, a remote village in Guinea that had been subjected to extreme forest depletion due to mining and lumber activity. Destruction of animal habitat meant that species and viruses hidden deep within forests now came into contact with humans more frequently, increasing the chances of animal to human virus transmission. The Ebola contagion went from Guinea to Nigeria and Mali, and via international travel to the West, spreading global panic.

Deforestation is not the only concerning issue. In 1992, Kent H. Redford published a landmark article in the journal Bioscience titled "The Empty Forest." It elaborated on how and why a seemingly healthy, large, and fully grown forest need not be so. A green forest seen from the air can be devoid of large mammals due to increasing human impact. The loss of large predatory mammals can create a species imbalance, reduce seed dispersal, and break the natural cycle. Trees with large seeds can begin to dominate the forest, disrupting the formerly balanced ecosystem of plants, animals, viruses, and bacteria, leading to unforeseen consequences.

There are, of course, those exceptional examples of human inhabitation within forests, while doing the least possible harm to them.

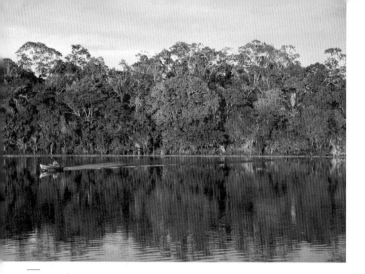

Figure 2.3
The Amazon rainforest at the Urubu river, Silves, Brazil
Source: Andre Deak (see Image Credits for details)

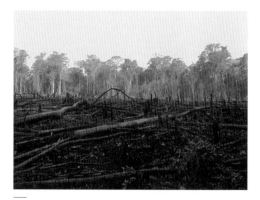

Figure 2.4
Forest depletion
Source: Dikshajhingan (see Image Credits for details)

The Korowai tribe of West Papua, Indonesia, for instance, live in tree houses 30 to 120 feet above the earth, offering them protection from the threats of the jungle below. Each tree house is inhabited for three to five years by groups of 10 to 20 residents, and a new home has to be built atop the tree on a cyclical basis. When the tree or area can no longer sustain the dwelling's construction, its location is moved to another jungle territory. This moving of the tree house is not just a matter of communal convenience. It is in fact a means for allowing the previous forest site to recover by letting trees grow back and giving nature a chance to heal itself. It is about ensuring that no permanent damage is done to any part of a forest through concentrated habitation. The exceptional dwelling pattern of the Korowai is as much about ecological regeneration as symbiotic habitation.

Such exceptions aside, contemporary urbanization trends, however well-intentioned, can have devastating effects on forests. In the mid-'80s, in response to population pressure, the ambitious Transmigration Program was initiated in Indonesia to help relocate people from densely populated inner islands such as Java to less populated outer ones like Sumatra. It was the largest voluntary land settlement effort in the world. The idea was noble but came at the price of destroying vast amounts of south-east Asia's forests, making these places some of the worst fire-prone areas in the country. Indonesia also offers another invaluable insight in this regard: In Sumatra, agroforests once under the purview of local rural communities have now been cleared for palm oil and paper factories. It goes to show that while controlled urbanization can help reduce pressure on forests by accommodating rural migrants in urban centers, the unchecked abandonment of rural areas can in fact trigger the widespread conversion of forests into areas for agriculture and industry.

The reverse, however, is also true - as seen in the remarkable reforestation efforts in Costa Rica. In the 1940s, tropical rainforests and indigenous woodlands occupied more than 75% of the country.

Between the 1940s and 1980s, uncontrolled logging led to severe deforestation, and by 1983, the country's forest cover had been reduced to a shocking 26%. Subsequently, new reforestation policies and programs were initiated. They include compensating landowners for reforestation and offering incentives for land protection through government grants funded through international donations and nationwide taxes. Land owners are allowed to extract only a certain number of trees from the forest and are simultaneously required to plant trees within deforested areas. After decades of commitment and implementation, the forest cover of Costa Rica has today increased to an impressive 52%, double that of the 1983 levels.

As we contemplate our future amidst the pandemic, we must not forget that urbanization and climate change will be two of the most important aspects that will shape our destiny in the decades ahead. They are deeply interrelated. On the one hand, our cities bear the potential to serve as engines of economic growth, particularly in the least developed countries, pulling millions out of poverty. But cities pollute the air, destroy living systems, pave entire ecologies with toxic slurries of gravel and oil, and insert thousands of synthetic chemicals into the environment. Each year, millions of acres of forest are turned into desert, and their inability to make rainfall via evaporation and transpiration means that large swathes of verdant lands are becoming drier terrains. Given that forests absorb vast amounts of carbon from the atmosphere, this will have significant implications for climate change and global warming. And this can transform the future of our cities with sea level rise, unpredictable weather patterns, resource scarcity, and pandemics.

In August 2020, an article titled "Current and future global climate impacts resulting from COVID-19" by P. M. Forster and his colleagues in the journal Nature Climate Change suggested that global greenhouse gas emissions had dropped 10–30% on average during April 2020 due to reduced human activity. But even if the pandemic were to last through 2021, these drops, the article argued, would not have much of a lasting effect on climate change unless nations incorporate "green" policy measures in their economic recovery packages. Per the 2019 United Nations Environmental Program Gap Report, which draws on the Intergovernmental Panel on Climate Change (IPCC) special report, global emissions in 2030 will need to be 45% below 2010 levels to limit warming. This means that they would need to fall by around 7.6% each year this decade to limit global warming to less than 1.5 degrees Celsius above pre-industrial temperatures.

This highlights the impact that intelligent policy and leadership will have on our collective future. It also reminds us that we urbanists need to be shoulder-to-shoulder with environmentalists in the campaign against global warming. If there is a side of this campaign that deals with the conservation and preservation of our forests, oceans and wetlands, then there is another that deals with the transformation of our attitudes to contemporary urbanization. This includes densifying existing transit corridors, upcycling abandoned industrial areas into new multi-use districts, rethinking urban policies that have perpetrated rampant sprawl, and limiting urban growth within inner cities without destroying the natural surrounds. It involves recasting our asphalted thoroughfares and parking lots as urban ecologies filled with trees, and transforming our toxic urban landscapes into gridded "forests" that breathe oxygen and prevent heat islands. And by designing our buildings with open-to-sky spaces that can nurture local flora, we can change our private domains towards greater ecological performance as well. The COVID-19 pandemic is an opportune time for us architects and urbanists to recognize that we too are environmentalists of sorts, with a crucial role to play in shaping our planet's future.

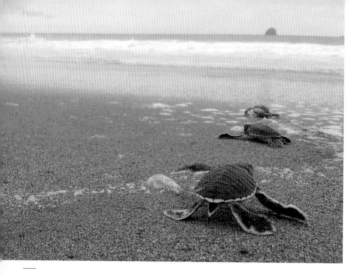

Figure 3.1
During the pandemic, due to the lull in human activity, thousands of turtles have hatched on barren beaches across the world.
Source: Iryanaraya (see Image Credits for details)

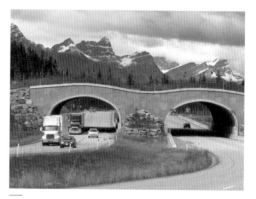

Figure 3.2
Wildlife overpass on the Trans-Canada Highway between Banff and Lake Louise, Alberta.
Source: WikiPedant (see Image Credits for details)

03

The Wild City

During the COVID-19 lockdowns, photographs of wild animals exploring our vacant cities have warmed our hearts. Cougars were spotted wandering the empty streets of Santiago, Chile. Wild goats descended from the hills into coastal tourist towns in Wales. Monkeys were scavenging trash bins for food in Lopburi, Thailand. Flamingos are flourishing in the lagoons along Albania's western coastline, where their numbers have increased by a third. In one of the world's busiest marine routes, the Bosphorus in Istanbul, Turkey, the lull in cargo and fishing boat traffic has attracted dolphins to the waters. The list goes on.

Such images are reminders of the degree to which wildlife has remained at the fringe of our mainstream city-planning discussions. Wildlife is even more marginalized than urban infrastructure, an aspect of our cities that is largely the domain of professionals focused on utilitarian concerns with no knowledge about the subtleties of ecological behavior. Little wonder that thousands of urban creeks, streams, and rivers lie mercilessly channeled, devoid of any life. Wildlife in the context of our cities remains the central concern of biologists and environmentalists, but their studies seldom find direct interface with architecture and city planning processes. For example, in their landmark 1998 article, biologists Michael Soulè and Reed Noss defined the idea of "rewilding" our cities. They posited, after patient observation and research, that large predators are often instrumental in maintaining the integrity of ecosystems and that they require extensive space and connectivity. They were calling for a more reflective outlook to how urban expansion and infrastructure intersects with biological behavior - identifying a major gap in our city planning practices.

There are some worthy efforts at this urban-wildlife intersection: In Canada, the Banff National Park is bisected by the Trans-Canada Highway (TCH), and to reduce the effects of this large arterial, 24 wildlife crossings (22 underpasses and two overpasses) have been built to ensure habitat connectivity while protecting motorists. The Netherlands boasts the world's longest wildlife overpass called the Natuurbrug Zanderij Crailoo. This massive structure, completed in 2006, is 50 meters wide and over 800 meters long and spans a railway line, business park, river, roadway, and sports complex. It also has over 66 wildlife crossings (including underpasses and eco-ducts) that protect populations of badgers, wild boar, and deer. As of 2012, the Veluwe, a thousand square kilometers of the Dutch region's woods, heathland and drifting sands, the largest lowland nature area in Northwestern Europe, contains nine eco-ducts, 50 meters wide on average, that shuttle wildlife across highways. And they also have reflector units called *wildspiegel* (wildlife mirror) to keep wildlife from crossing motorways at night.

More significantly, these efforts are monitoring the actual workings of these built structures to understand their effectiveness. Since 1996, Parks Canada has collaborated with researchers to consistently assess the success of the crossings. The past decade has produced a number of publications (for example Clevenger & Waltho, 2000, 2001, 2007) analyzing the crossings' impact on various species and overall wildlife mortality. Per Clevenger's 2007 analysis, 10 species of large mammals (including deer, elk, black bear, grizzly bear, mountain lion, wolf, moose, and coyote) have used the 24 Banff crossings a total of 84,000 times as of January 2007.

The research has also identified how wild animals need time to adapt to such structures before they feel comfortable using them. Per Parks Canada unpublished results, grizzly bear crossings increased from seven in 1996 to more than 100 in 2006, although the number of bears using the structures remained the same. Wolf crossings increased from two to approximately 140 over the same 10-year period. Similar monitoring is currently underway in the Netherlands as well. In short, these projects stand out for their willingness to embrace their potential shortfalls and improve on them.

While such efforts embody a sensitive attitude to urban wilderness, they also draw our attention to the resilience and adaptability of wild animals to everything we impose on them. They suggest that the contemporary city is getting increasingly "wild." For instance, the howls of coyotes have managed to reach midtown New York, and they have responded to decreases in their population levels with an increase in their reproductive rates. Canada now has a new species, the Coy Wolf, a hybrid from coyote and wolf parents with the best qualities of both, lurking along Toronto's freeways and using these less inhabited routes to navigate the city.

Meanwhile, peregrine falcon chicks are hatching atop Brooklyn Bridge and Boston's skyscrapers fulfilling the bird's natural preference for cliffs and mountain peaks. Tokyo researchers have observed crows dropping scavenged walnuts on highways so that moving cars can crack them open. Pigeons are roosting under Puerto Rican eaves undaunted by urban contamination. Gangs of Rhesus Macaques have made historic buildings in Jaipur their domain. Stork chicks are hatching atop London's chimneys. Feral cats are overcrowding Rome. Squirrels are crossing Los Angeles streets on telephone cables. Manhattan summer nights are being filled with choruses of insects competing with car alarms and garbage trucks. Birds in Mumbai have learned to make nests of worn-out shirt hangers amidst the paucity of twigs.

And now, during the pandemic lockdowns, with our diminished human activity, nature and wildlife is pushing back even more. The question therefore is: How do we bring these ecological aspects into our mainstream discussions on city making? As professionals and activists focused on our built environment, we urbanists have a consequential role in answering this question. By incentivizing public transit in place of cars, encouraging urban infill over suburban green-fields, "foresting" our cities, and working with ecologists to replenish degraded ecosystems, we can reverse the attitudes and trends that have marginalized wildlife within our cities and pushed it into the diminishing corners of the planet.

There are three kinds of "wilderness" when viewed from the city today. The first is wilderness in its original form, encompassing the wealth of our rivers, forests, wetlands and all the biodiversity they nurture. The second is the tortured and abused wildlife within our cities. It includes numerous denizens that, far from being extinct, have desperately adapted to a forest of another kind - where thoroughfares are canyons and skyscrapers are cliffs. The third is the wildlife in our rewilded cities where streets and highways are eco-corridors, and where parks and greens are not just places for human recreation, but designed ecologies where pollinators of all forms can flourish and thrive.

This notion of rewilding our cities is only part of a bigger vision that the eminent wildlife broadcaster David Attenborough has described as rewilding the world. In his insightful recent film, A Life on Our Planet, he offers an explanation of what we can do to once again live in balance with the natural world. It includes halting deforestation, bringing back wilderness, and enabling animals on land and in the sea to repopulate to sustainable levels. It means cutting off our reliance on harmful and unsustainable fossil fuel and stabilizing human populations across the world by providing universal healthcare and pulling people out of poverty. Attenborough words are hard-hitting: "The world is not as wild as it was. Well, we've destroyed it. Not just ruined it. I mean, we have completely...

well, destroyed that world. That non-human world is gone. Human beings have overrun the world."

As we digest the pandemic crisis from a human perspective, we must recognize the significance of the thousands of turtles that have hatched on barren beaches in Thailand, and the wild boars that have been spotted in the empty streets of Barcelona. Such images serve to remind us of our essential role as stewards of a "multi-species urbanism," a term first coined by artist-researcher Debra Solomon in her essay "Soil in the City: The Socio-Environmental Substrate" (Solomon and Nevejan, 2019). It describes urban development framed by natural world concerns, to "promote policy innovation for natural world stewardship, recognizing humans as participants within a more-than-human habitat." Such practices, on the one hand, are about reclaiming and conserving wilderness, and on the other, about augmenting the wilds through the design of responsive socio-ecological landscapes that mitigate human-animal conflict.

Our cities are complex multi-species ecologies, and urbanism, as a professional discipline, a science, and an art, is at its best, an empathetic, multi-species endeavor. A truly sustainable, inclusive city can never be about environing humans alone.

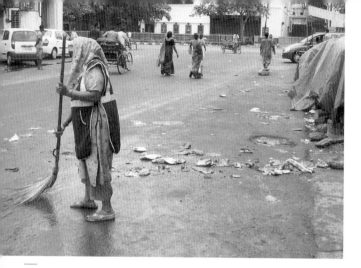

Figure 4.1
Street Sweeper, New Delhi, India.
Source: Author

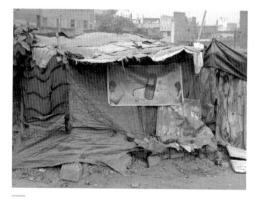

Figure 4.2
Temporary squatter dwelling made of canvas and other gathered material, New Delhi, India
Source: Author

04

The Unfair City

Heartbreaking images of rural migrants in India fleeing cities to return to their villages, of families with children walking on foot, have shown us the degree to which this pandemic affects us all differently. Following the impositions of the COVID-19 lockdowns, thousands, forced out of jobs and with no means of earning a daily living, have been left with little choice. As we endure the harsh impacts of the pandemic, those that are being hit the hardest are the millions of underserved with no access to adequate housing. For them, the "safe at home" idea is meaningless. As United Nations chief António Guterres noted in a recent address, the impacts of the pandemic are falling "disproportionately on the most vulnerable: people living in poverty, the working poor, women and children, persons with disabilities, and other marginalized groups."

We live in unjust, unfair cities. We are the ingredients of a socio-economic system that is not able to treat everyone equally. How wonderful would it be if the right to the city was equitable for one and all? If the wealth of public places, access to jobs, and privilege of easy mobility was available to everyone, irrespective of social class or income level. But this is not the case. All cities have economic polarizations, some more stark than others, and between them is a mundane middle that sustains both extremes. The nuances of how these extremes negotiate the middle, is what the shaping of an affordable, or in turn, unaffordable city is all about.

The unaffordable city has various global guises. Singapore is one of the most expensive cities in the world, whose livability quotient is synonymous with an impeccable cleanliness and urban order. Per 2020 rankings, Paris is even more expensive, where modest-paid workers have had to take up illegal and substandard rooms, even as the poor and elderly are carted out to the urban edges. And in Tokyo, with the Fukushima disaster prompting a shutdown of all 50 nuclear reactors across Japan, residents are paying more than ever in household electricity bills.

Meanwhile, with nearly 50% of Asia's and Africa's populations becoming city dwellers, and more than 75% of Latin America already there, inner city poverty is one of the biggest challenges of our time. With infrastructure hardly developing at the same pace as the largest and fastest-growing cities in Africa, Asia, and Latin America, the demographic bulk fueling this growth has to live in temporary shelters and slums. Weak ownership rights leave slum residents economically vulnerable and unable to build safe, sturdy houses, and these habitats consequently become easy victims to weather, fire, and crime. Lack of safe, clean water means that families often have to buy it at high prices from vendors. Inadequate sanitation and waste disposal leads to disease. And illness means loss of livelihood, leaving families struggling to buy food.

There is a deeper environmental consequence to all this. Urban poverty endangers the lives of millions and the unhygienic conditions their habitats generate also damages streams, wetlands, and rivers. And environmental degradation continues at an even bigger scale through middle- and upper-class over-consumption and increasing industrial production, both of which damage natural resources. Even as the poor are denied access to fundamental infrastructure, governments are financially unable, or even averse to investing in efficient systems. The challenge of the polarized city is as much environmental as political, and as much about social justice, as human psychology.

How can we make the city more equitable for everyone? Where do we begin to bridge the ends of urban inequality? Numerous ongoing bottom-up practices and campaigns by activist and non-government organizations to grapple with extreme issues can never be underestimated. But the unaffordable city has many broader dimensions as well - rampant sprawl, inefficient mobility, rising home prices, air pollution, and the destruction of nature. These issues are compromising the long-term viability of our cities for both the rich and poor and everyone in between.

For example, there is a direct relationship between affordability, walkability, and transit. In the United States, the least afford-able cities are born out of a gross disconnect between housing and transportation costs compared to one's household income. Because North American cities have sprawled into vast automo-bile-dependent places fed by highways, malls, and job centers, the less-affluent have to commute long hours for work, spend more on gas, and pay more taxes. On the other hand, New York City and San Francisco have relatively high housing costs, but they also rank among the lowest-cost cities for transportation, because they are designed to facilitate walking, along with an extensive and heavily used mass transit network. In cities with the dire need for bridging polarized extremes, the answer does not lie at the extremes, but in between.

Curitiba stands out in this regard. By 1960, this Brazilian city's popu-lation had increased within two decades from 120,000 to 361,000. Even as planners were contemplating widening roads for more cars, Curitiban architect and planner Jaime Lerner took office as mayor in 1971. He introduced dedicated bus lanes along the city's main arteries, with stations placed in medians. The intent was to allow buses to run at speeds comparable to light rail, while dramatically reducing the cost. Lerner made a bargain with private bus opera-

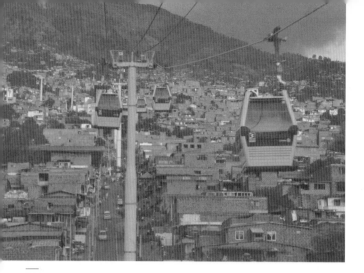

Figure 4.3
The Metrocable system, Medellin, Colombia
Source: Jorge Láscar (see Image Credits for details)

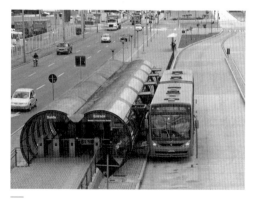

Figure 4.4
Bus Rapid Transit system, Curitiba, Brazil
Source: Mario Roberto Duran Ortiz (see Image
Credits for details)

tors to pay for the new infrastructure in exchange for the vehicles, thereby reducing the cost of the bus lanes to 50 times less than rail. The first line opened in 1974, and by 1993, with new routes added, it was carrying 1.5 million passengers a day. Today, the Rede Integrada de Transporte has 157 bi-articulated and 29 single-articulated vehicles and is used by 2.3 million passengers of all income levels and class each day, representing 85% of Curitiba's population.

Bogota, Columbia is another case in point. On becoming the mayor in 1998, Enrique Penalosa hiked gasoline prices, and poured revenues into putting public space and public transit at the forefront. Inspired by Curitiba, the TransMilenio bus system was introduced and given the best space on the city's avenues in exclusive lanes, making cars and minibuses secondary. The sleek red look of these buses, and the use of high-quality finishes for the bus stations also helped boost its status. The TransMilenio began to move people of all income levels so effectively that general commuting times across the city plummeted, and by extension, people got heathier.

In Medellin, Colombia, there is a 385-meter-long escalator installed in one of the city's poorest sections called Comuna Trece. It opened in 2011. More than giving residents access to the city, it has provided the city's institutions access to one of its remotest areas. Consequently, the municipality, nonprofits, police, and housing corporations have been able to improve public services, bring in housing improvement subsidies, create social programs for children and young mothers, and help the younger demographic resist temptations of gang involvement. Medellin also has a cable car system called the Metrocable operationally integrated into the rest of city's mass transit network. It provides transportation to hilly areas with underdeveloped barrios that are inaccessible by the city's mass transportation system. Since its opening in 2004, it carries over 30,000 people on a daily basis. Medellin's escalator and cable car system have neither directly ameliorated the physical conditions of the underdeveloped settlements, nor reduced the city's overall income inequality. But for the first time, residents of the city's

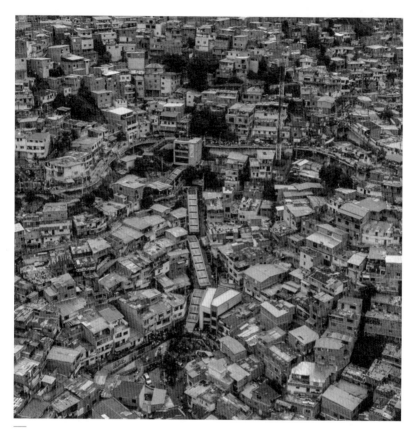

Figure 4.5

A 385-meter-long escalator in Medellin, Colombia, installed in one of the city's poorest sections called Comuna Trece, gives its residents access to the city

Source: Juan Gómez (see Image Credits for details)

poorest neighborhoods feel a real connection to the city and vice versa, giving both a greater sense of belonging.

When it comes to affordability and affordable housing, there is something we can all learn from the social housing organizations in the Netherlands. These non-profit foundations own roughly one third of the country's total housing stock, and function like a non-profit mutual credit card company backed by the government - making it easier for them to close loans with banks for low interest rates. Due to this, they can not only afford to keep rents low, but build projects wherein it is hard to differentiate between the social housing component versus the other. Families with low income are not only assured that their landlord will charge them a just rent, and their houses will be well maintained, but also that there will be no social stigma associated with one's level of income. As such, the Netherlands is a country where the affluent and less privileged reside in the same neighborhoods, send their children to the same schools, and buy their daily needs at the same stores.

The cases discussed above are neither perfect nor radical. They are simply sincere, practical efforts that have redistributed the city's benefits to make it fairer and more accessible to the largest number of people, and through their own specific means. The pandemic is currently widening the urban divide that has resulted from our long-term failure to address basic human rights. In a post-COVID-19 world, we must strive even harder to find ways of providing all urban residents housing and healthcare, so that everyone can live with dignity and be prepared for the next global crisis. In this light, if the cases discussed above affirm anything, it is that investing in our cities to help people feel more equal is not just about making our cities equitable and just, but also stronger and resilient.

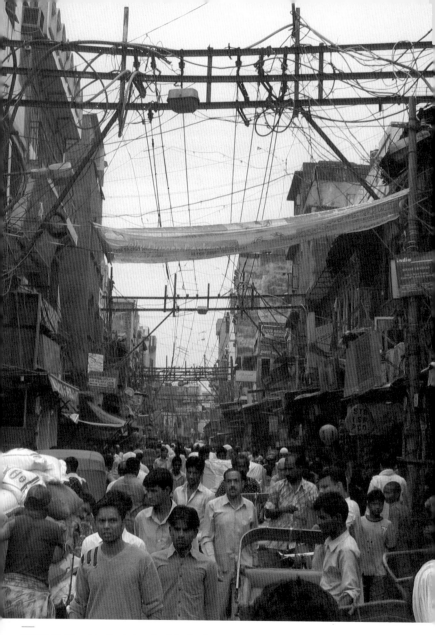

Figure 5.1 **Street in Shahajanabad, India.** Source: Author

05

The Informal City

As of 2020, per the International Labor Organization, over two billion people, constituting more than 60% of the world's employed population, are earning their livelihoods in the informal economy - that is, commercial activities occurring outside a governing body's observation and regulation. The informal economy supplies our cities with a vast labor pool - from housemaids to street vendors to rag pickers - for the many "unpleasant" jobs that organized labor continues to evade. Because these denizens need to work on a daily basis to earn their livelihood, lockdowns and other containment measures stemming from this pandemic are exacerbating their vulnerabilities. On the one hand, they are susceptible to greater health and safety risks due to inappropriate protection measures. On the other, they have no guaranteed access to medical care, employment benefits or income security were they to fall sick. For members of our informal economy, the pandemic is a double-edged sword.

The relationship between the informal economy and our cities is a dominant subject in urbanism and architecture today. Aspects such as slums, squatters, urban villages, bazaars, street food, roadside vending, and hawking are being increasingly recognized for the uncanny entrepreneurship and economic resourcefulness of the underprivileged, and also as counterpoints to the notion of the city as

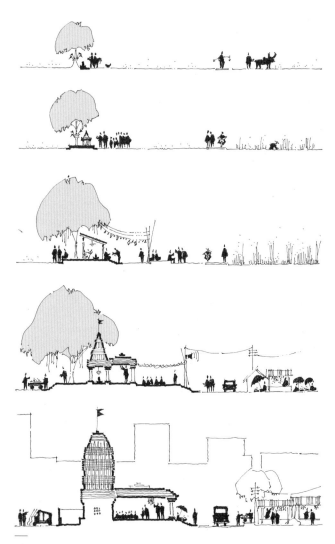

Figure 5.2
Evolution of an anonymous wayside shrine into an urban temple.
Source: Author

a formally organized, and policy-driven entity. Scholars like Alonso Ayala and Vinit Mukhija have focused on the informal city with studies of inadequate urban housing. Others like Rahul Mehrotra have observed the city's "kinetic" aspects, as repositories of local wisdom. Some like Nihal Perera have studied spaces created by ordinary people, as victims in the cities that marginalize them.

My studies have focused on informal spaces that blur the boundaries between the public, private, and sacred - for example, the consecrated urban tree, typically marked with banners or sacred insignia along an urban street. The space beneath the boughs of such a tree often serves as an informal gathering place for street hawkers and unhoused denizens, not unlike the *chaupal* (platform under a tree) in the center of an Indian village. Such trees have significant bearings on the future of the Indian city, for many of them have historically seeded the makings of some of India's largest temples, and even entire temple towns.

The notion of tree worship is born out of the ancient Hindu philosophy of an omnipresent divinity. Shading a smeared stone or marked with thread, flags, and banners, a *devasthana* (place of the deities) appears mysteriously under a tree's branches, bearing the spiritual weight of an entire community. When a positive change happens, the tree is endowed with gifts as a mark of gratitude, and its increasing eminence gradually elicits its transformation into a wayside shrine. When the tree dies, the spot continues to remain sacred, believed to be vibrant with the energies of innumerable rituals of worship.

Many wayside shrines grow over time into rudimentary temples. They become identifiable urban markers, typically endowed with communal sponsorship with minimal infrastructure, such as electricity and water, and an assigned priest or caretaker. The Pipaleshwari Kali Mandir in New Delhi, for instance, is located near Connaught Circus in the city's central business district on a vacant lot. Beneath a peepul tree are multiple statuettes housed within a shed-like structure. There is a modest chamber for storing the temple's daily apparatus. Bells hang beneath the eaves. A metal board in the branches advertises the temple's scope of religious services. At around six o'clock each morning, a maintenance lady sweeps and washes the space around the shrine. A snack vendor and a barber set up an open-to-sky shop. A couple of cycle rickshaws park nearby waiting for customers. A wandering hermit who has made this shrine his local destination for over 20 years appears on his rounds. By seven in the morning, a priest dressed in saffron garb prepares the place for daily rituals before worshippers begin to arrive.

Many such modest shrines evolve further into franchised Hindu temples, completing the sacred spot's maturation from simple anonymous beginnings to legitimate ownership. This is a millennial pattern of informal Indian urbanism. For example, the Meenakshi Temple in Madurai, one of the largest temples in India, is said to have evolved from an anonymous stone *lingam* (symbol of the deity Shiva) under a tree in a forest around 1600 BCE, morphing into the vast complex it is today, through centuries of communal worship, patronage, and craftsmanship. Beneath the branches of thousands of consecrated trees within the Indian city then, lie the seeds of an informal urbanism that we cannot afford to underestimate. Size does not matter; what matters are the locations of these sacred dots powerful enough to bypass socio-economic legitimacy and exert powerful influences on Indian urbanity. Today's consecrated trees will become tomorrow's centers and monuments. In them lie the hopes and spiritual aspirations of the millions of underserved, who generate and nurture our informal economies, and who are simply claiming their stake in the city.

Our empathy for this demographic has never been more important than now, during the pandemic. We need to identify, embrace, and include them in our efforts and initiatives more urgently than ever before. We need to give them a voice. This is a moral issue that must seek to bridge the socio-economic injustice this crisis has revealed.

It is also a practical one, because our cities rely so much on the skills and abilities of the members of the informal sector, that we cannot function efficiently without them. The impact of this pandemic on their lives is serious and significant. In Uganda, vendors have resorted to sleeping in markets so that they can continue to earn a living while avoiding contact with their families, and in numerous cities - from Los Angeles to Accra - street hawkers have reported a 90-percent drop in their income due to reduced foot traffic during the lockdowns.

There are, however, some inspiring reports. In South Africa, food vendors were given permission to trade during lockdown measures, with concurrent safety guidelines by public health authorities to minimize the pandemic's spread. In Barcelona, street vendors joined forces with a local clothing company to sew masks and aprons for health workers. In Malaysia, street vendors found ways to work during the lockdown with a drive-through and pick-up service. And in Washington, D.C. they partnered with the city to become public health ambassadors to curb the spread of the virus.

Such observations highlight our professional limits as designers, architects, and planners. How do we engage with the informal forces that shape our cities? How do we negotiate our spatial and aesthetic preoccupations with the uncanny creativity of the informal city? The fact is that we architects and planners, with our intellectual pursuits, are but one among numerous other actors shaping the city. Thus, while the increasing scholarship on the informal sector is not only essential but thoroughly revealing, the typical tendency to pit the informal city in opposition to the formal methods through which cities are being made is, I would argue, to miss the point. The formal and informal aspects of the city do not exist in isolation. They coexist, collide, negotiate with, and sustain each other every day.

Urban informality is a barometer to gauge the engagements and negotiations we franchised designers make with the formal city. It

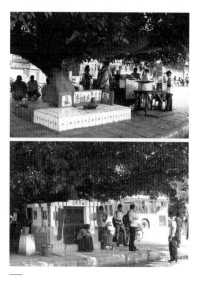

Figure 5.3
Evolution of a sacred insignia under a tree into a small shrine in New Delhi, India
Source: Author

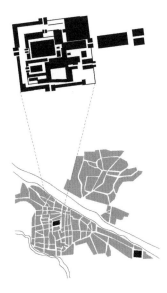

Figure 5.4
Evolution of Meenakshi Temple in Madurai, India, from a simple shrine into a large sacred campus surrounded by a city
Source: Author

is a lens to better understand the diversity of situations and needs in our cities and guide our most influential entities such as politicians, administrators, and policy makers. One of the things we designers can do amidst this pandemic is open conduits to working directly with social solidarity organizations, particularly those already active in the informal economy, and help augment their responses to the situation we all find ourselves in.

This means that the fields of urbanism and architecture must expand their sphere of concern to help create places that care for and protect the ingredients of the informal city. If urban informality is about creativity and entrepreneurship, how can urbanism and architecture help augment and celebrate such aspects? If it is about marginalization and economic polarization, how can we help mitigate such aspects?

What this eventually boils down to is the idea of urbanism not as a high-art but an act of high-activism. As professionals equipped with skills to design built environments, our role as advocates for social justice can never be underestimated. We architects and urbanists can be the bridge between the formal and informal city, if we can be modest enough to recognize where and when to assert our opinions and where and when to let go. The informal and formal city are not opposites, just as poverty and prosperity need not be seen in opposition. They are, as Nihal Perera has noted, altering conditions and multiple realities that inevitably and simultaneously make up our cities. We must engage seamlessly with them, and on their own terms, toward bigger goals of social and economic justice. This is what making inclusive cities is truly all about.

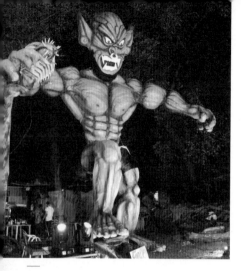

Figure 6.1
Narakasur (demon) effigy in Goa, India,
during the annual Diwali festival
Source: Siddha Sardessai

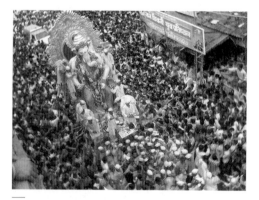

Figure 6.2
Statue of the Hindu deity Ganesh being paraded
in the streets of Mumbai, India, during the annual
Ganesh Festival, before it is immersed in the sea
Source: Ninadism (see Image Credits for details)

The Privilege of Community

The World Health Organization has appropriately corrected our use of the term "social distancing" to "physical distancing." While it is absolutely essential to maintain physical distance from each other during the COVID-19 pandemic, it does not mean that we socially disconnect from our family members and loved ones. But even so, physical distancing must feel like a punishment for humanity. It is in opposition to our fundamental nature of being with and around each other in various capacities, for various reasons, in various places. Thanks to digital media, we can work, meet, and discuss things. But the beauty of the casual, informal, even accidental human interaction is one of the things we have lost in this period. The pandemic has awoken our caution radars and taken away our spontaneity. Our cities have lost the magic of the human crowd, of publicness, of community, and we are impatient to claim it back.

We gather in our cities for many reasons, but the crescendo of such cohesions are our numerous festivals. We come together during festivals for no other motive than to glorify a collective idea linking our past to our future, making it different from a demonstration or casual gathering. As the most enduring cultural blueprints of a place, the physical enactment of our festivals in public space is therefore a shared privilege we can never take for granted.

Consider for instance Diwali, Hindu India's archetypal festival. In my native city, Panaji, in Goa, something magical happens during this festival each year. Each neighborhood, precinct, locality, building complex, or micro-community is represented by a Narakasura (demon effigy symbolizing evil) in various forms and sizes enabled by communal contributions. Their specific locations offer clarity on the perceived territorial boundaries of various communities otherwise difficult to trace within the urban matrix. Preparations begin weeks in advance - first a skeleton of bamboo or metal, then a buff body of hay and old clothes stuffed with firecrackers, followed by a coat of thick glued paper and oil paint, and, finally, a meticulously made papier-mâché face. Narakasura is the much-awaited annual offspring of a Goan Diwali, only to be burnt and destroyed at the crack of dawn.

In the southwestern regions of India, three months prior to the Ganesh Festival in August, artistic clay models of the deity, varying anywhere from an inch to over 25 feet, are made for sale by skilled artisans. The festivities begin with the installation of small Ganesh statues within homes, and larger ones within the public domain housed in temporary structures called *pandals*. On the eleventh day, the statues are paraded through streets and immersed in the sea - symbolizing a ritualistic send-off to the deity on his journey toward his abode, taking with him the misfortunes of his devotees.

The idea of a public domain free for the populist expression of hundreds of erected Narakasuras, or the massive religious processions of the Ganesh Festival, is testimony to the unique workings of an urban engine. Events like these are not just performances of religious ritual, but annual experiments in community management and civic pride. For example, during Diwali, houses and entire complexes are decorated with lights and lamps, and cultural activities are accompanied by public singing, theater, and orchestra performances. There are philanthropic activities like free medical checkups, blood donation camps, and charity for the underprivileged. There is economic exchange, with people buying new clothes, gifts, and artifacts, with malls and stores well stocked, and with street vendors, taxis, and rickshas all remaining busy. Be it the Carnaval gathering in Venice, the Saint Patrick's Day parade in Ireland, or the Harvest Moon celebration in China, festivals are cultural catalysts that recharge our cities and communities with a renewed social and economic energy.

How are such events playing out in the COVID-19 world? The Gion Matsuri, one of Japan's most famous festivals held in July in the city of Kyoto, was cancelled in 2020 due to the pandemic. Ironically, the festival had an even greater symbolic significance in 2020, because its origins trace back to an epidemic in 869 CE. Kyoto was founded in Enryaku 19 (by Western count 800 CE, the year of Charlemagne's coronation). A hundred years after the capital had moved from Nara to Kyoto, a plague spread throughout the city killing thousands of people. The crisis was seen as an expression of the gods' anger toward humans not living a clean and hygienic life. The emperor petitioned for rituals to appease the *kami* (spirits). It included the use of 62 *hoko* spears each representing one of the country's provinces, along with parading the main deity of the Gion Shrine (now Yasaka Shrine) to purify the city. While some may argue that the Gion Festival ought to have been celebrated on an even grander scale to pray for the expulsion of the pandemic just as it did centuries ago, concerns of the coronavirus spreading obviously took precedence.

Meanwhile, Holi was celebrated on March 9, 2020, in several states across India with people wearing masks as they smeared color while avoiding mass gatherings. In Sevilla, Spain, in late March, the city's streets normally crowded with ornate Semana Santa (celebration of Holy Week leading up to Easter) processions and floats, were eerily quiet, with people celebrating in the confines of their homes. In Japan, for Kyoto's annual Aoi Matsuri held on May 15, the colorful procession that attracted thousands of spectators in 2019 was cancelled. However, Shinto priests gave offerings at the Shimogamo Shrine and prayed for peace and an end to the pandemic. In late August 2020, the Brihan Mumbai Municipal Corporation (BMC) introduced a "one-ward-one-idol" concept to ensure social distancing measures during the Ganesh Festival celebrations. More than 35,000 police personnel were deployed across the mega-city to ensure that the ritualistic immersion of the Ganesh idols remained incident-free. In 2020's mid-November's Diwali celebrations, Narakasura effigies were distinctly fewer in Goa, and public gatherings were limited across India, but cityscapes glittered as much as the previous year to commemorate the "Festival of Lights."

We adapt, not just to new and changing circumstances, but also to new insights on the impacts of our habits. Over the past decade festivals in India, for instance, have become increasingly conscious of their environmental implications. The bursting of crackers during Diwali has seen a decline to keep the air more breathable. During the Ganesh Festival, awareness of environmental pollution caused by the immersion of thousands of idols has instigated changes. Since the idols are made from non-bio-degradable Plaster of Paris, they continue to float, choking water bodies and adversely impacting the aquatic ecosystem; and they are often decorated with toxic lead-heavy paint adding further to this issue. Consequently, eco-friendly Ganesh idols made from red soil, some even containing plant seeds, are now becoming increasingly popular.

Urban festivals remind us that our cities are the repositories of our memories, crucibles of our cultural inheritance, and threads to a precious past that we are not willing to let go. Our patterns and rituals of community life and publicness evolve and mature over time because they are as much a psychological as a physical phenomenon. Being public, private, communal, or aloof is a choice we all have. One could be sitting in a public plaza surrounded by like-minded people yet lost in a private conversation on a laptop screen. Or one could be dressed in formal attire from the waist up, within the private boundaries of one's bedroom, and be engaged in a public discussion via digital media.

In the COVID-19 world, the idea of community will find new definitions, stemming from both our behavior patterns and the manner in which we use our public spaces. Physical distancing, the increasing reliance on digital technology, and even the frequency with which we choose to be in public may all appear to challenge our preconceptions of what being communal, public, and private means. Amidst all this, we must not fail to realize that even though the specifics of our public patterns may be forced to change, this pandemic is a temporary phenomenon. We must adapt, improvise, and innovate within these strange circumstances. But we must never forget that our instinctive urge to engage in publicness, and be part of a community, is a choice, and therefore a privilege we will always have.

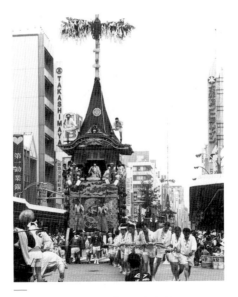

Figure 6.3 **Gion Matsuri parade in Kyoto, Japan.** Source: Noboru Asano

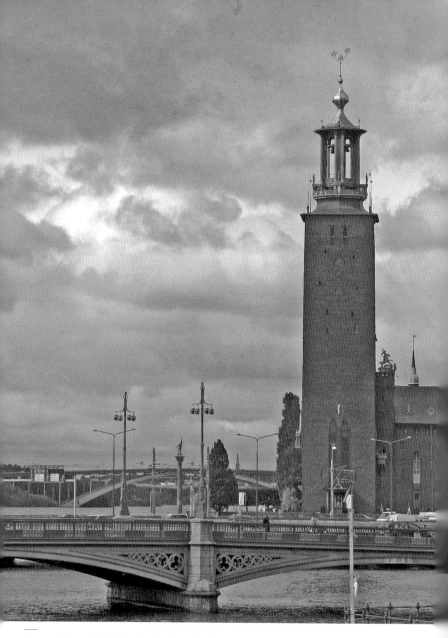

Figure 7.1 **Town Hall, Stockholm, Sweden.** Source: W. Bulach (see Image Credits for details)

Governance Matters

In a strange way, the pandemic has united humanity toward a common concern. No matter what our cultural or geographical differences may be, we are together in riding through this sudden global crisis. Yet, the specific attitudes, responses, and actions of our leaders, administrators, and citizens toward the pandemic have also highlighted how diverse we are as contemporary societies. It has shown that our cities are different not because of the way they look, but because of the way they are governed and administered.

Consider for instance the idea of participatory planning, a privilege many of us, particularly those living in democratic societies, take for granted. That concerned residents can opine publicly, initiate proposals and provocations, present them to administrators and elected leaders, and expect them to be heard, is something many cities across the world simply do not have. This is the privilege of shaping the urban future together through inclusive, communal dialogue and negotiation; in contrast to a city being shaped exclusively by those with power and influence, or by unequivocal authority.

Of course, the specific workings, expectations, and outcomes of democratic planning and public participation themselves are quite different across societies and nations. The most obvious difference is the acknowledged role and place of the public voice within the larger framework of public policy. In the United States, for example, public participation is a legally mandatory part of the city planning process. Among other things it was the Standard Zoning Enabling Act in 1926 published by the United States Department of Commerce that initiated language requiring public notice and access to hearings. It stipulated that no regulation, restriction, or boundary would become effective until a public hearing was held where citizens would have an opportunity to be heard. The law also required citizens to be given at least 15 days of notice regarding the time and place of such a hearing. Many nations and cities outside the United States have no such mandate. The perceived accountability and trust associated with public officials and the track record of such deliberated exchanges is consequently different in different societies.

There is a direct relationship between the modes of everyday urban governance and regulation and the visible experience of a city. In the United States the planning and policy milieu is a decentralized landscape in that every city is an independent jurisdiction with the authority to craft its own zoning policies and planning ordinances. In Pasadena, where I reside, a low- to mid-density multi-family housing project has to be mandatorily designed around an open-to-sky courtyard. The same project would be illegal in the neighboring city of San Marino whose zoning code does not allow multi-family housing at all. The same project in the city of Santa Barbara's urban core would have be designed only in the Spanish-Revival style. The urban planning landscape of the United States is like a series of independent kingdoms, each sustained by their own rules. Different cities, all shaped through participatory planning processes, can still function differently because of their policy and entitlement process specificities.

Cities also look different because of the invisible policies and processes that shape them. For example, in the United States, sprawl and its accompaniments, however much we may despise them, are entirely legal, because zoning codes have allowed the separation of uses, permitted wide thoroughfares fronted by impervious parking lots, and buildings with blank walls to the street. In turn, North American cities have reversed sprawl by reversing the regulations that have perpetrated it. Thanks to visionary initiatives by public officials and leaders who are willing to change petrified regulations, competent professionals who are willing to advocate beyond business as usual, and, most importantly, thoughtful citizens who are willing to support these ideas for the greater good of their city.

In China, unlike the United States, most development rules are crafted at the national level, and negotiating changes to these codes at a local and regional level is very difficult. The only exceptions to this are the "Special Economic Zones" (the equivalent of "Free Zones" in the United Arab Emirates). These are areas with greater local jurisdictional authority and more relaxed regulations with the objective of offering tax and custom-free benefits to attract expatriate investors. The impressive skylines of Shenzhen and Pudong are embodiments of this. The intentions behind urban regulations thus directly influence urban form. Which is why Hong Kong, China's plot ratio (a development's total built area divided by its total site area) is similar to New York's downtown district ranging between 6 and 10. But it is significantly higher than London (1 to 6) or Shanghai (1.6 to 2.5) or Singapore (2.2 to 4).

The bridge between the visible city and the invisible processes sustaining it, is at its best a participatory, collaborative engagement between visionaries and enablers. If visionaries are immersed in the front-end creative intelligence, then enablers are the equally important follow-through engines. A municipality's efforts in negotiating existing rules to enable an exemplary project is as visionary as a progressive plan within tight budgetary and spatial constraints. Designers may not always be the visionaries, and municipalities not always the enablers. This indeed is one of the shifts that is continuing to transform cities today. The gradual, yet vivid transformation of sprawled downtowns and main streets into walkable places, the recasting of zoning regulations into vision-based codes, the transformation of suburban malls into compact urban mixed-use destinations, and the conservation and renewal of urban ecosystems and rivers are as much about progressive municipal vision, sound follow-through and citizen support.

But all this said, how does one ensure that the positive effects of our well-intentioned policies can reach people that need it the most, particularly during this pandemic? Per the International Rescue Committee, people in refugee camps in Bangladesh, Syria, and Greece face a heightened risk of COVID-19 due to more densely populated conditions. As such, the more difficult aspects of urban governance are about being able to cater to the underserved demographic whose colossal, dense, informal settlements make physical distancing during this pandemic anything but easy - and this is particularly significant in cities in Asia, Africa, and Latin America.

An insightful article titled "COVID-19 Pandemic and Informal Urban Governance in Africa: A Political Economy Perspective" in the Journal of Asian and African Studies recently argued that while the pandemic is a pervasive health problem, it should also be recognized as "a social and political economy challenge." The article argues for networks that interconnect entities in state and local governance, the private sector, the civil society, and the informal sector toward common goals. The authors see the pandemic as an opportunity for city authorities to rethink their engagement with people living in informal settlements by recognizing the potential of non-state entities to help transform urban governance.

Numerous such entities - from humanitarian foundations to non-government organizations to citizen initiatives - are already at work to support populations hit by the pandemic. In Pakistan, the nonprofit organization Shaheed Syed Ali Raza Abidi Memorial Foundation (SSARA) is delivering freshly cooked meals and grocery packets to members of the transgender community. The UK-based organization Total Giving is raising money to help Rohingya communities with packages that include face masks, soaps, and vitamin supplements. In Lucknow, India, the Sangraha - Mask of Need initiative is helping to support local artisans by having them embroider masks to meet their basic needs. And in Nepal, CARE's Emergency Surge Fund is distributing soap and water, and installing handwashing stations to protect the most vulnerable.

The pandemic has highlighted the degree to which such simultaneous urban initiatives can actually reach places and people in our cities where municipal policy may not. It has shown us that our cities are multi-layered socio-political ecosystems with many protagonists - civic leaders, public administrators, private practitioners, and, most importantly, numerous other non-state entities who are doing incredibly consequential work on crucially important issues. It has underscored the importance of cooperation and coordination among different levels of governmental and sectoral institutions.

The COVID-19 pandemic is a litmus test that will reveal the degree to which our respective local, regional, and national leadership can use this unprecedented time to rethink its place and role in the complex network of effective urban governance. As the pandemic wanes, we will all need a boost of assurance and confidence when it comes to aspects like healthcare, emergency preparedness, affordability, and economic stability - particularly those that have the least voice. Will our cities and societies be able to overturn the pandemic from crisis to opportunity, and not just learn from our previous shortcomings but act on them toward a more just future for all? A sincere broadening of our urban governance network, to include the many other on-the-ground grassroots entities within our cities will go a long way toward this.

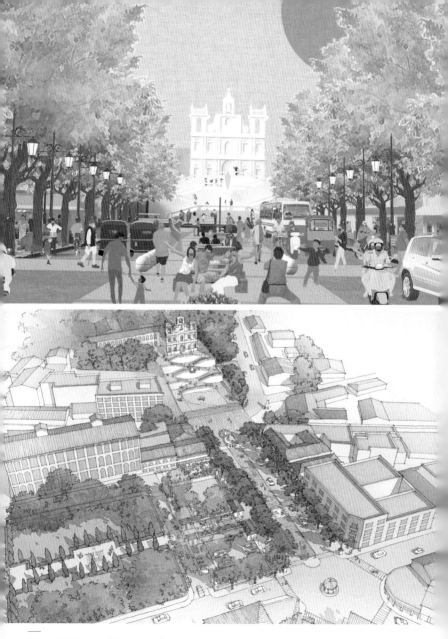

Figure 8.1 **Proposal for upgrading Panaji Church Square, Goa, India, by Vinayak Bharne & Siddha Sardessai, circa July 2021.** Source: Author

08

Paradigms of Open Space

It has become increasingly evident that the COVID-19 virus is mainly transmitted through extended close contact, particularly in enclosed spaces, through the accumulation of droplets and aerosols. A crowded, air-conditioned grocery store or hospital has a greater possibility of spreading the virus than a park or street. This means that it is our plazas, streets, courtyards, terraces, roof-gardens, and patios - indeed the combined urban network of open-to-sky spaces - that will foster the social malleability we need during these testing times. Inviting open spaces at all scales encourage people to use them. Their lack in turn encourages us to stay indoors. In a broader sense, the pandemic has simply underscored the crucial importance of intelligent open space design - public, semi-private, and private.

Public open space throughout human history has been about both the container and contained, and more perti-nent to this pandemic is the design of public spaces as urban lungs with fresh air, sunlight, and landscape according communal activity with adequate distancing. One thinks of the 120 x 90-meter Plaza Mayor in Madrid (circa 1619) where the dense surrounding fabric is randomly cut off, because the plaza is literally carved out of them. The open-to-sky rectangle is defined by a four-sided building "frame" that mediates the adjacent streets with arched openings. At the 560 x 160-meter Naqsh-e Jahan Square

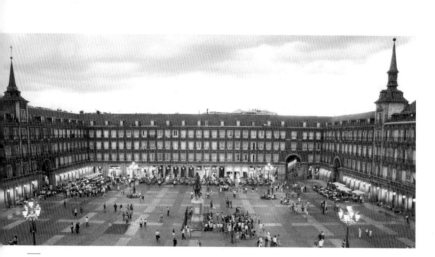

Figure 8.2
Plaza Mayor, Madrid, Spain.
Source: Sebastian Dubiel (see Image Credits for details)

in Isfahan (circa 1600), a former polo field, the disparate uses of a palace, two mosques, and a market are unified with continuous walls and arcades. And though the 4 x 0.8-kilometer Central Park in New York (circa 1857) looks like a natural landscape, it is in fact a major engineering feat, having removed more than 10 million cartloads of material, and planted four million trees and shrubs.

But large public spaces are not always within the city. In 1837, William Light proposed Adelaide Park, a vast 930-hectare figure-eight-shaped open space that today separates the City of Adelaide from the surrounding metropolitan region. And Kyoto in Japan has a public space larger than any of the mentioned examples. The mountains that envelop the gridded city were humanized in the sixteenth century by siting temples and monasteries transforming them into a colossal natural public garden.

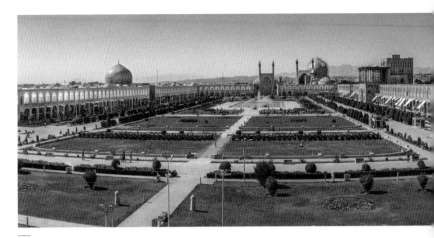

Figure 8.3
Naqsh-e Jahan Square, Isfahan, Iran.
Source: Arosha-photo (Reza Sobhani); (see Image Credits for details)

Our most ubiquitous public space, however, is the street, and with the pandemic outbreak, the lack of indoor activity in restaurants and theaters is increasing attention to this adjacent public domain. Numerous tactical interventions are reconfiguring the street as an adapted public space. With lower traffic volumes, the surplus space of the asphalted travel lanes is being reclaimed for outdoor dining while practicing physical distancing. New York City, for example, has pedestrianized two streets per neighborhood to decongest sidewalks and augment physical distancing. This is not a new concept. Back in 1976, the city of Bogota in Colombia introduced the Ciclovia program under which select city streets became car-free on Sundays and holidays between 7 a.m. and 2 p.m., generating a 585-kilometer pedestrian, and bicycle-only open space network.

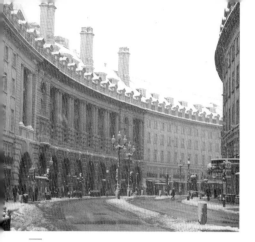

Figure 8.4
Regent Street, London, United Kingdom
Source: Jon Curnow (see Image Credits for details)

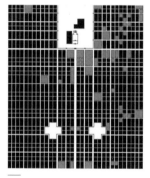

Figure 8.5
Original plan of Kyoto, Japan
Source: Author

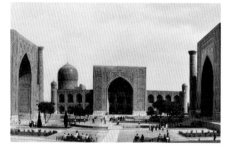

Figure 8.6
Registan Square, Samarkhand, Uzbekistan
Source: LBM1948 (see Image Credits for details)

Then there is the concept of "Privately Owned Public Space" (POPS) stemming from planning policies designed to incentivize the creation of public spaces using private capital. In Japan, for example, where buildable land is scarce, there are national POPS standards to incentivize developers. By negotiating deals beneficial to both sides, new open spaces - from sidewalk extensions and plazas, to arcades and through-block passages - are built by private entities, with covenants allowing them to be accessed by all. In return for providing these, developers are given opportunities to increase revenue, generally though greater building area or tax cuts. The idea was first introduced into New York City's zoning regulations in 1961 and has resulted in over 590 POPS at over 380 buildings within the city, providing over 3.8 million square feet of additional public space - equivalent to roughly 10 Central Parks. On June 27, 2020, the New York City administration temporarily suspended certain zoning requirements for Privately Owned Public Spaces (POPS) to enable retail establishments and commercial buildings to reopen after the COVID-19 lockdown. The idea was to increase the amount of outdoor space to enhance physical distancing.

The specifics of how we use open spaces are, however, regionally and culturally diverse. While the plaza, piazza or square represents the traditional public space prototype in the Western world, its equivalent has never quite flourished in pre-industrial south and east Asia. Looking at plans of traditional cities such as Changan, Nara, and Jaipur the most prominent public spaces are the main avenues structuring the city and leading to the palace complex. The rest of the city is a grid of tenuous streets punctuated by local landmarks such a temples, and it is in these linear spaces that rich public life - from markets to festivals - has traditionally flourished. From Regent Street in London to Registan Square in Samarkhand, the use of public spaces has always been rooted to the cultural signatures of their respective worlds.

Our cities today also have other public space distinctions. For instance, Mumbai has merely 1.1 square meters of public space per person, compared to 31.68 square meters in London and 26.4 square meters in New York. Public spaces in cities like Mumbai - from cricket fields and beaches to parks and streets - serve a complex web of social and economic functions, making them vibrant and spontaneous on the one hand, and crowded and chaotic on the other. During the pandemic, the required semblance of organization - from the six feet distancing rule to linear queues - has forced public spaces in cities of the global south to adapt and generate new patterns of publicness.

Another emergent COVID-19 open space paradigm is outdoor classrooms in schools. They respond to some of the challenges of providing in-person instruction with physical distancing guidelines. They help expand access to in-person instruction, especially for disadvantaged students for whom the remote learning experience has been less than ideal. Not to mention the value that being outdoors brings to a child's social, emotional, and mental wellbeing. Of course, outdoor classrooms are easier done in places with moderate than extreme climates. Yet the poetic image of children being imparted knowledge under the boughs of a tree than within a closed building seems to hit hard during these times. One thinks of Finland's "forest schools," where kindergarten and pre-school age children spend up to 95% of the school day outdoors in the wilderness exploring, playing, and learning about the world around them. It began in the 1950s, when Nordic schools introduced a morning walk into the daily routine and it became the highlight of the children's day. While the rest of the world moved toward a results-based curriculum, Scandinavian teachers observed the positive effects that nature walks had on young students and forest schools grew in popularity.

Which brings us to another demographic, the elderly, who are not only more susceptible to the coronavirus, but also cannot venture far from their dwellings - highlighting the need for open spaces within our residential enclaves. It wouldn't be unfair to say that at the scale of the individual building, mainstream development has reduced private open spaces to balconies and terraces associated with an individual unit, but there are some progressive examples in this regard. In 1989, the city of Pasadena in California adopted the City of Gardens Ordinance, wherein a multi-family building is required to have a "garden rectangle" with specific planting requirements. This is essentially a revival of the traditional courtyard housing dwelling type wherein individual dwellings are arranged around open-to-sky spaces, giving all units a shared garden. As density increases, units get attached and partially stacked around single or multiple court-yards, that become shared outdoor living rooms complimenting the public spaces of the city.

This said, open spaces during this pandemic are but one of the pieces of a far more complex urban puzzle wherein millions of people across the world who do not have a home, and who live on streets are being left to fend for themselves. In some places like Ethiopia, in April 2020, a day after declaring a five-month long state of emergency, the government began initiatives to rehabilitate thousands of homeless people to prevent the spread of COVID-19 among those living outdoors. But numerous others whose daily work activities have come to a sudden halt face a dubious future. In our efforts to adapt our cities to this pandemic we cannot afford to forget those that are being affected the most.

New paradigms of open space may stem as responses to the looming pandemic, but their lasting value will lie in their ability to bridge extant social injustices and economic inequalities. The pandemic then is a trigger to revisit what inclusive open space design truly means. The intelligent (re)design of our public, semi-private, and private open spaces can be one of our most effective means to ensuring that no one in our cities is left behind.

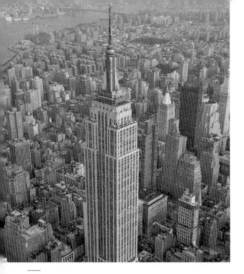

Figure 9.1
Lower east side of Manhattan.
Source: Sam Valadi (see Image Credits for details)

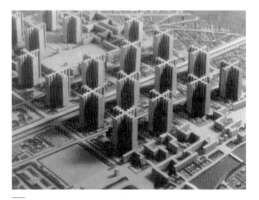

Figure 9.2
Model of the Plan Voisin for Paris by Le Corbusier displayed at the Nouveau Esprit Pavilion (1925)
Source: SiefkinDR (see Image Credits for details)

Rethinking the High-rise City

New York City, along with Wuhan and Milan, were among the hardest COVID-19-hit cities during the 2020 lockdowns. They share the common trait of high-rise, high-density living, a paradigm in which New York has historically played the most prominent role. Going through two of the earliest high-rise construction booms in the world, the first before 1910 and the second between the mid-1920s and early 1930s, New York City today ranks third globally in the sheer number of high-rise buildings, only after Hong Kong, China and Shenzhen. These three cities direct our attention to one of humanity's greatest architectural accomplishments - the high-rise building - which has come into a new light during the pandemic.

The urban fabric of Manhattan in New York, is a careful assembly of high-rise buildings that define streets and open spaces. Principal avenues carry buildings taller than the side streets. Mid-block alleys carry service uses behind the buildings allowing consistently positive street frontages. When New York's 1916 zoning ordinance required buildings to step back to allow ample light into the street space, numerous Art Deco towers, in response, used a fairly planar 10 stories to create a street face, beyond which towering, pinnacled masses strove upward to create the skyline. Manhattan offers invaluable lessons on how the collective arrangement of individual high-rise buildings can generate something wonderful and bigger than themselves.

It was precisely this image of Manhattan that Le Corbusier famously compared with his alternative version of "the Contemporary City" in his 1924 book, The City of Tomorrow and its Planning. His new model depicted an airy field of 24 cruciform skyscrapers standing within a park. The street grid was replaced by a field of gigantic mega-blocks, and the tower redefined as a freestanding object. Le Corbusier went on to demonstrate this model's application by superimposing it on the traditional grid of Paris. In response to what he saw as the congested, unhealthy traditional city, his "Plan Voisin" erased the historic horizontal fabric centered on courtyards imposing a new urban order. The project was never realized, but the model and its manifesto - eventually known as the Ville Radieuse - marked a turning point for the formal, social, and moral dimensions of city making.

Central Business Districts now became galleries of new high-rise models. Popularized by New York's Lever House (1952), towers had their own plazas linked exclusively to private interiorized office parks. As seen in John Portman's hotels, glazed towers perched on brutalist podia accommodated parking and service uses with dead street faces. With developers vying for maximum land value, the high-rise building became a popular production housing proto-type, erupting randomly within finely grained traditional neighbor-hoods regardless of adjacencies. This blatant extrusion - the direct result of a linear Floor Area Ratio (FAR)-based zoning that estab-lishes a buildable area maximum per site - is now synonymous with high-end production housing from Buenos Aires to Mumbai.

The most dramatic products of this FAR syndrome are the "circum-stantial hyper-Manhattans" of Southeast and East Asia. Tokyo's fragmented, cacophonic spurts of high-rise buildings have resulted from ad hoc piecemeal vertical extensions of historic lots by succes-sive entrepreneurs. As seen in Roppongi or Kachijo, high-rise build-ings are surround by low medieval fabrics, creating sharp disjunc-tions right next to each other. In Hong Kong, China, with individual property owners competing for optimum land value, peculiar fabrics of tall thin buildings on small traditional lots have erupted with little concern for light and air. These "pencil skyscrapers" have an extremely low aspect ratio (gross floor area divided by the number of stories) compared to typical high-rise buildings in the United States or Europe. They are 20–25 stories in height with a floor typically containing no more than a pair of 400-square-feet units, with the bottom two floors dedicated to commercial use.

With the pandemic outbreak, high-rises across the world are being viewed from a new perspective. Issues like faulty plumbing, poorly circulated air, increased contact with high-touch surfaces, and the inability to engage in social distancing practices are raising caution. A century ago, in 1918, when the influenza pandemic claimed the lives of over 30,000 people in New York, Manhattan's population dropped from nearly 2.5 million in 1920 to 1.5 million in 1970, and we may be witnessing a similar phenomenon today with droves of people escaping to the suburbs and smaller cities. Some argue that this population dispersal will spread jobs and reduce housing costs. But over time, this could also repeat the worst mistakes of suburban sprawl, particularly the rampant development of the natural countryside, and the increasing reliance on the car. And while people in New York have the choice of moving to the outskirts, others in places with limited buildable land like Hong Kong, China and Tokyo do not.

Cities like Seoul and Taipei that contained the coronavirus in 2020 succeeded in doing so not by separating people but by increasing testing and monitoring people-to-people contact. If we look closely at the densities in New York, we find that COVID-19 cases in 2020 were concentrated in the outer suburban areas such as Brooklyn, Staten Island, and Queens - highlighting the difference between population density versus building density. It suggests that neither low suburban nor high inner-city densities necessarily relate directly to transmission risks. The chance of being infected is far greater in a busy retail store than a high-rise building adapted for the pandemic. We have learnt that the coronavirus is mainly transmitted through extended close contact, particularly in enclosed spaces, through the accumulation of droplets.

While we must remain cautious about concentrated population density, we must not be averse to high residential density in our cities. The two are very different. The former refers to the amount of people, the latter to the number of residential units, within a finite land area. In the United States of America, per the 2012 census, the most densely populated urbanized area - Los Angeles/Long Beach/Anaheim area in California, with nearly 7,000 people per square mile - is a low- and mid-rise fabric. The New York/Newark area has an overall density of 5,319 people per square mile, compared to Mumbai's 83,660 people per square mile, and Manila's 119,600 people per square mile.

These facts have significant implications for urban design and planning, for it is these disciplines that can adapt our cities to avoid the syndrome of concentrated population without losing the virtues of high residential density. Concentrating or dispersing people has to do with the design of public and private spaces. It is our parks, plazas, and patios - indeed the combined urban open space network - that will determine the quality of our gathering patterns during this pandemic period.

In turn, high residential density does not necessarily translate into a high-rise city. A high-rise building within a single parcel can achieve significant densities of over 100 dwelling units per acre, but on a large parcel, the separation of multiple high-rise buildings to allow sufficient light and air lowers their cumulative density, needing them to be taller. Taller buildings are not only expensive but also cut off their residents from the ground plane of the city. In fact, the intelligent hybridization of seven-, four-, and three-story buildings on a single parcel can itself achieve close to 100 dwelling units per acre. Cities like Amsterdam and London embody this idea.

Some of the finest social housing projects in recent decades from the global south not only demonstrate the virtues of the low-rise, high-density model, but also offer another crucial lesson in light of the pandemic: In societies where air-conditioning is simply too expensive a proposition, the very form of the dwelling unit and building must foster cross-ventilation through natural means. This is where a single-loaded corridor building allowing air to flow through each unit, is far superior to a double-loaded corridor version, or high-rise tower with a central core with no natural air circulation. The high-rise building as an architectural prototype thus has its demerits and will need to be adapted for the pandemic. Improving its air quality filters, ensuring that its plumbing is up to code, reducing the number of high-touch surfaces in common spaces such as elevators, and installing handwashing stations, are all measures that should not be underestimated.

High-rise buildings adapted for COVID-19, may be the dominant prototype for cities with extremely limited land resources. But for those that do have a choice, the mid- and low-rise, high-density model is certainly a better option, not just due to lower construction cost, but greater and easier access to common open spaces with fresh air, sunlight, and nature for families, children, and the elderly. What we truly need during this pandemic is a critical examination of various dwelling types and their density potentials, along with deeper examinations of the numerous other elements of our urban landscape that are inextricably related to our buildings.

Living in our cities is not about shelter alone. It is about having access to mobility, public space, and multiple aspects that supplement our private residential patterns. High-rise or mid-rise, it is the intelligent integration of the myriad elements constituting our cities that will determine our urban destiny as much as the thoughtful design of our dwellings themselves.

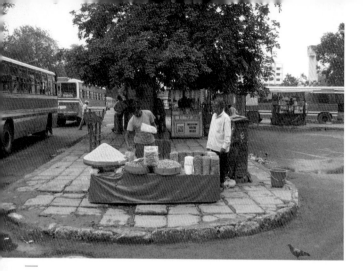

Figure 10.1
Street hawkers (New Delhi, India) create innumerable centers that formal planning does not account for
Source: Author

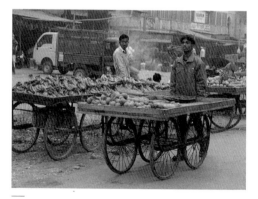

Figure 10.2
Fruit vendor with mobile cart, Varanasi, India
Source: Author

10

Shaping the Polycentric City

The pandemic and the lockdowns have localized our daily physical world. We do not want to venture too far from our homes. During the confinement, we have been forced to realize the simple benefits of the "polycentric city" - wherein multiple centers within walking distance of our neighborhoods can become the basic armature around which our cities are shaped.

The polycentric city is part of our urban inheritance; all pre-industrial cities were planned this way, and there was a practical reason for it. Before automobiles and trains, animal-driven carriages and human feet were the only means of commute. Distances could not afford to be vast, and habitats had to be compact. Thus, the hamlet, town, and city, however culturally different, followed the common idea of being walkable - to and within. With the advent of industrial inventions, cities expanded into vast urban landscapes. In places like Los Angeles, whose explosion was catalyzed by an impressive train network, the lure of the automobile resulted in something terrible - the organized dismantling of•the trains and their replacement with freeways slashing through historic neighborhoods and districts. Epitomized by the North American post-war suburb centered on the indoor mall at its heart, the polycentric city had been replaced by a new model where places devoted to exclusive uses now relied on the automobile as their sole connector.

The demerits of such toxic models had not gone unnoticed. In early 1900s, American urban planner Clarence Perry proposed an alternative based on a theoretical proposition by the urbanist Lewis Mumford, that he disseminated through the 1929 Regional Plan of New York and its Environs. The basic idea was to design a neighborhood or district as a compact pedestrian shed with a ¼-mile radius, the number referring to a maximum distance an average American walks, typically lasting five minutes. The center of the shed had the community center and school, with shops at the neighborhood edge. But as the Neighborhood Unit concept spread across the globe, it also began to interiorize and disconnect communities. For example, in Ashdod, Israel (circa 1956) the vast industrial area was supplemented by 17 introverted neighborhood units each with 10,000 to 20,000 people, resulting in a decaying commerce center between.

In the 1990s, town planners in the United States such as Andres Duany revisited Perry's original Neighborhood Unit and offered some astute rectifications. They created multiple street connections between adjacent neighborhoods replacing Perry's original idea of surrounding a neighborhood with highways. Since a neighborhood demographic outgrows the use of the central school as children become adults, the new version of the neighborhood unit, called Traditional Neighborhood Development (TND), has retail and community amenities in the center with the school moved to the outskirts between multiple neighborhoods. There is also a gradient of dwelling types, from denser buildings in the center and less dense ones at the edge. And in the most recent iteration called the Sustainable Neighborhood Unit, espoused by urbanists such as Doug Farr, the spaces surrounding the pedestrian shed are storm-water-retention playfields and habitat corridors, adding a crucial environmental dimension to the model.

The notion of a polycentric city had also been suggested from a multi-cultural perspective in Christopher Alexander's seminal 1977 book, A Pattern Language. In pattern 8, titled "Mosaic of Subcultures," he posited the idea of breaking the city into a vast ensemble of different subcultures, each with their own spatial territory and "small enough, so that each person has access to the full variety of life styles in the subcultures near his own." Rather than seeing the city as homogeneous expanse of buildings, streets, and open spaces, Alexander's model is composed of community precincts based on common backgrounds or cultural histories, the largest being "as much as a quarter of a mile" with 7,000 residents.

The good news is that the polycentric model is already at work in many of our cities today. Even automobile-dominant metropolitan areas like Los Angeles have seen significant shifts with individual cities reviving their downtowns as new local centers, and mixed-use regulations replacing Euclidian zoning codes. In cities across North America and Europe, where policy and regulation enabled single-use sprawl - not accidentally, but through planned, legal means - the conscious reversal of these very urban policies is now enabling the polycentric city model to re-emerge at various scales.

In this re-emerging polycentric model, an important catalyst is transit nodes, from train stations to bus stands, where people gather in large numbers. Imagine how incredible our cities would be if we were to make such nodes well-designed destinations with beautiful plazas and streets, energized with a rich mix of retail, office, and residential uses. People living next to these transit nodes would rely less on their cars and be incentivized to use transit to go from place to place, particularly if it is affordable, efficient and of high quality. This is what the Transit Oriented Development model, a well-worn rubric in city planning today, is all about. Tokyo works exactly this way. An impeccable train network connects multiple transit nodes from Ginza to Shinjuku to Akihabara each with their distinct identities, making it one of the greatest polycentric mega-cities in the world.

Japan has a far more important lesson to offer in this regard, and it has to do directly with zoning. Japan has only 12 basic zones, far fewer than a typical North American city. The zones are organized per their degree of nuisance. Unlike the United States, where each zone is limited in what uses can and cannot be permitted, zones in Japanese cities are less exclusive with low-nuisance uses allowed everywhere. For example, a factory cannot be built in a residential neighborhood. But housing can be built in a light-industrial zone. There are rules to guide how tall and dense residential buildings can be in various parts of the city, but the principal idea is that almost all Japanese zones allow a mix of uses, which naturally enables a poly-centric landscape.

Cities in the global south are already polycentric - albeit in an unplanned way. The vast urban informality of vendors, street hawkers, and wayside shops that situate themselves at the fringe of neighborhoods and along important avenues, despite being illegal, create innumerable centers that formal planning does not account for. The result is strangely magical: One's daily needs are available within the proximity of one's house, even though the city's planning instruments did not intend for it to be this way. The question in such cities - from Mumbai to Phnom Pehn - is not so much about changing planning policy as it is about creating the mechanisms to accommodate and make a place for the many entities that are rendering a polycentric landscape in the first place. This means rethinking the design of our city's public spaces, and rede-signing our streets to create organized space for vendors, based on a careful study of how their daily patterns actually work. It means efficient garbage collection and street cleaning to ensure these zones remain hygienic. It means balancing reinforcement with tolerance to enable urban informality to thrive without letting it go beyond a tipping point.

This brings us to another important aspect of our daily needs - food - and its relationship to our inner cities in the form of urban farms and edible gardens. In Cuba for example, urban farms produce over 65% of the country's food on only 25% of its land. The trend started in response to the 1990s economic crisis when lack of food imports instigated local food production. In 2016, 300,000 urban farms generated 50% of the national fresh produce, including fruits, vegetables, meat, and eggs. Close to 100,000 backyards and 5,000 plots, along with rooftops and balconies, grow fruit and vegetables with the surplus given to schools, hospitals, and universities at subsidized prices.

The shaping of a polycentric urbanism suggests numerous shifts in aspects that currently make our cities - zoning, urban form, neighborhood structure, public transit, public space, informal activity, food production, and more. And while the polycentric city as a post-COVID-19 urban model reassuringly has global value, the paths to getting there will have to stem from on-the-ground socio-political realities within our respective locales. The transformation of our post-industrial cities from single-use, automobile-dependent landscapes into mixed-use, multi-centric ones will depend as much on our individual initiatives as those we demand from our leaders, administrators and policy makers. Hopefully soon, this pandemic will be a thing of the past. And by then, the merits of the polycentric city - getting to know your neighbors and local vendors, driving less, and walking more - will not just be epiphanies and realizations, but new habituations that we practice and advocate everywhere.

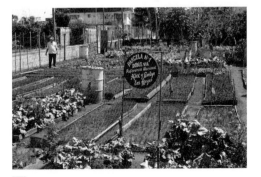

Figure 10.3
Urban agriculture, Havana, Cuba. Source: Arnoud Joris Maaswinkel (See Image Credits for details)

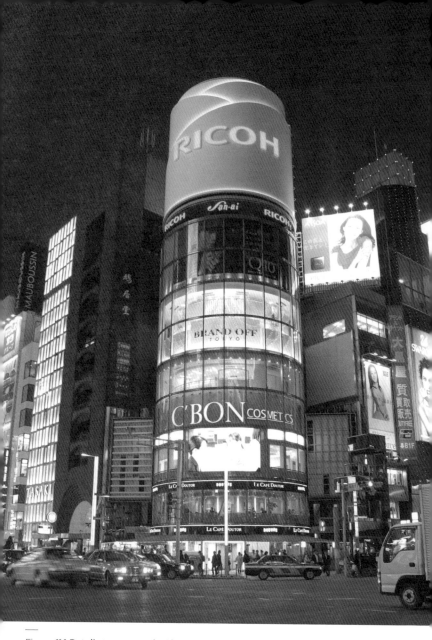

Figure 11.1 **Retail streetscape in Ginza, Japan.** Source: Author

11

Rethinking Retail

The pandemic has affirmed how much we consume our cities. It has changed the way we look at our daily needs and instigated rethinking on how little we need compared to how much we spend. This has had an immediate impact on the retail industry, and with restaurant dining and shopping in indoor malls coming to an abrupt halt during the lockdowns the impact on non-essential retail such as non-food and fashion products has been particularly severe. Customers have remained focused on essential retailers, while retailers in turn have responded with no-touch practices such as curbside pickups and home deliveries. Amidst numerous store closures, employee furloughs, and the psychological impact the lockdowns and physical distancing have had on us all, the retail industry as we know it may see a new normal in the coming future.

What this simply means is that the retail industry will have to reinvent itself once again. It will have to generate new experiences to lure customers within the realities of the pandemic. This is not a unique thing. Retail across the world has always been an experiential phenomenon constantly adapting to changing consumer tastes and market trends. For example, over recent decades, across the United States, regional indoor mega malls have increasingly fallen victim to failed retail chains and changing demographics. Shifting customer tastes prefer outdoor shopping and dining,

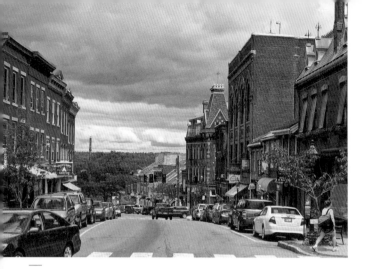

Figure 11.2
Historic Main Street, Belfast, Maine, United States
Source: Bruce C. Cooper (see Image Credits for details)

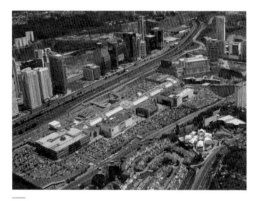

Figure 11.3
Centro Santa Fe mega mall, Santa Fe, Mexico
Source: Serge Saint (see Image Credits for details)

despise freeways and grid lock, and crave the character and quality of enduring places. Consequently, these large, multi-block sites with vast parking lots have been reclaimed and restructured as outdoor "lifestyle centers" organized around plazas, parks, squares and streets to cater to the changing market.

This is a direct critique of retail trends that transformed the traditional city. In Los Angeles for example, from the 1920s to the 1950s sweeping changes began to reconfigure retail environments prioritizing size over any pre-war urban precedent such as main streets and squares. Mammoth regional complexes began to expand the scope of merchandise for specialty outlets and large department stores to serve the growing residential areas outside the historic downtown. In 1927 Sears opened its immense 425,000 sf building. In 1928, Bullocks Wilshire opened a 200,000 sf department store with a 375 car motor court. In 1951, the 26-acre, 3,500-car Sears Valley Plaza Store pioneered the realigning of buildings away from the street to front the car lot as the new secret to the retail precinct's vitality. Two decades later, the Shopping Center at Century City inverted priorities with multi-level car parks below and a pedestrian "piazza" above. In the '80s the Beverly Center built eight stories of almost blank plaster walls along an entire city block, and in 1996 AMC opened the largest mega-plex in the nation - a 30-screen, 5,700-seat theater at the Ontario Mills Mall under the pseudonym of "interactive shoppertainment."

As counterparts to historic retail centers, such examples across the world not only reinvented the retail experience to center on the use of the car, but also physically transformed the city by creating retail mega-blocks that evenly dispersed space for buildings and cars. A number of traditional urban patterns were consequently transformed: Mixed-use districts were replaced by single-use destination projects. Pedestrian-scaled street grids became car-dominated mega-blocks. Commercial and retail places began to be designed as monumental buildings. And, the pattern of buildings collectively

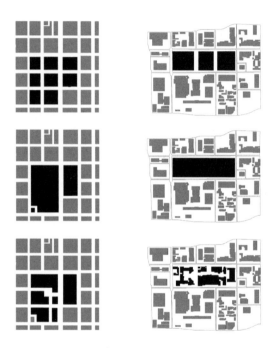

Figure 11.4 (Left) Evolution of CityPlace, Long Beach, California (Right) Evolution of Paseo Colorado, Pasadena, California. The original city grid (top); the mega-mall that disrupts the grid (middle); and the new grid that accommodates retail anchors and housing (bottom). Source: Author

defining streets and open spaces was replaced by parking domi-nated self-referential projects that had little to do with their adja-cencies.

It is against this backdrop that one must appreciate the degree to which new retail trends centered on pedestrian-scaled blocks, streets and buildings have recast the retail experience in recent decades. According to Ellen Dunham-Jones of the Georgia Institute of Technology, of the estimated 1,500 enclosed malls built across the United States since 1956, around 1,000 are still being used for their original purpose, while 500 have closed or changed to a different use. Of these, 56 have been rebuilt as mixed-use urban places, with another 75 proposed to be transformed into mixed-use destina-tions. The "malls to mixed-use centers" idea has had an impressive track record across the United States: from Mizner Park in Florida, City Centre in Texas, Santana Row in California, and Mashpee Commons in Massachusetts. They have housing accompanying retail and office uses, transforming the stereotypical image of the mega-mall into a vibrant mixed-use town-center. These projects are not mega-buildings, but human-scale, street-friendly develop-ments that re-establish the traditional relationship between the urban grid and the public realm.

How might the retail experience change in the COVID-19 world? For obvious reasons of safety and hygiene, the focus on essential items, reduction of shopping visits, pick up without stepping into the store, and the use of credit cards and phone payments over cash are all becoming increasing popular. But the most signifi-cant change unfolding amidst the pandemic is the accelerated reliance on online shopping. E-commerce giants such as Alibaba and Amazon are reshaping the retail terrain. Amazon hired 175,000 new employees during the pandemic. And it is expected to invest heavily on pandemic-related expenses such as getting products to customers and keeping employees safe. Clearly, the pandemic has highlighted the important role digital technology will play in the everyday life of retail consumers across the world.

What impact might this have on the design of cities? On the one hand, trends such as curbside pick-ups and drive-through delivery suggest an increasing reliance on the automobile. This could have a devastating impact on cities, due to car-dominated streets and less-pedestrian activity - reviving the early 1900s' debacles of car-centered urbanism. On the other hand, the lure to spend time away from being locked at home can inspire a renewed investment in reshaping our public spaces so that customers can enjoy the urban outdoors while practicing physical distancing - and this is already happening.

For instance, streets in the historic downtown of Pasadena (called Old Pasadena) in California have converted on-street parking lanes into outdoor dining spaces directly fronting restaurants, thereby allowing greater space for physical distancing. But there is another important lesson Old Pasadena offers us about transforming the relationship between parking and public space. The success to revitalizing this formerly blighted historic district was the idea of "Park Once." This means one parks one's car in a spot and walks to various retail stores instead of parking within lots at each destination within the district. While this may sound much like parking at a shopping centre, the vast asphalted mega-mall parking lot is now replaced by a series of city-owned parking garages, and the indoor mall is replaced by a real, vibrant open-to-sky street. Old Pasadena's city-owned garages are located within walking distance of all the retail destinations and provide 90 minutes free parking. The garages are not only designed to be compatible with the historic buildings but also have a street-level building liner with continuous retail along the sidewalk making the walking experience seamless.

Retail design in the COVID-19 world may also entail the frequency with which retail appears within the urban fabric. Retail nodes can be situated in ways that enable people to walk to them from their homes relying less on the car or even mass-transit. This translates into a variety of retail places of various types, sizes, and capacities within and around our neighborhoods. It means decentralizing retail and luring customers to take short walks or drives from their houses to enjoy the outdoors while shopping for essential items rather than making online buying the only option. Needless to say, this model also has environmental and health implications. Less driving means cleaner air. Walking more means a healthier lifestyle. And if we want to get even more progressive about it, increasing concerns about the global food supply can inspire initiatives for local businesses to grow food within their communities and neighborhoods, further reducing the carbon-footprint.

The pandemic has instigated serious re-thinking on our retail habits, trends, and priorities. While retail may be one of the most important economic drivers in our cities, we have now come to see it strictly beyond our individual conveniences for the many other aspects of our life it impacts. The debacles of the past century offer us numerous cautions about conceiving the retail experience and its physical environments in isolation, as if they do not affect anything else. As we adjust to our changing lifestyles during the pandemic, we must remember that the transformation of the retail experience from traditional mixed-use streets to indoor single-use mega-malls and back to outdoor mixed-use centers was in large part a reaction to our shifting priorities. At the end of the day it is *we*, the consumers, that wield the power to shape the retail experience in the post-COVID-19 world.

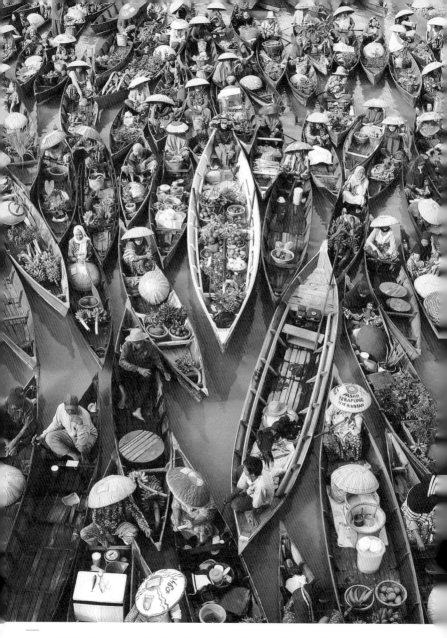

Figure 12.1 **Floating market in the village of Lok Baintan, South Kalimantan, Indonesia.**
Source: Muhammad Haris (see Image Credits for details)

Saving Vernacular Urbanisms

Even before the COVID-19 pandemic outbreak, more than 800-million people across the planet have been grappling with another serious global crisis - the lack of access to clean water. But unlike the virus behind the pandemic, the reasons for the water crisis vary significantly across climatic and geo-political boundaries. They range from issues of extreme water scarcity in arid regions to those of inefficient infrastructure and inadequate distribution even in places blessed with abundant rainfall. From villages to megacities, millions across the world struggle to access water for drinking, cooking, cleaning, and growing food.

With the pandemic outbreak, the gravity of the looming water crisis is becoming even more pronounced. An insightful recent paper titled "COVID-19 pandemic as a further driver of water scarcity in Africa" by Alberto Boretti has elaborated on why the pandemic "has dramatically changed the time frame" of the water crisis. The pandemic coupled with a suffering economy, is shifting priorities from ensuring water and food availability to all. Due to the lockdowns, people in several parts of the world are unable to leave their homes to access water even as they lack the financial means to purchase it.

This not only highlights the socio-economic inequalities we have generated as societies, but points to the limitations

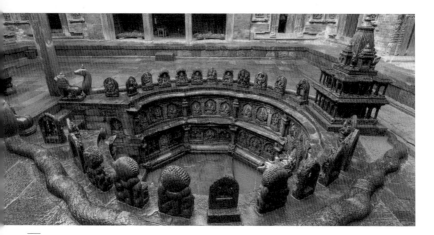

Figure 12.2
Tusha Hiti, Patan, Nepal
Source: Bijaya2043 (see Image Credits for details)

of industrial technology in meeting the demands of our crowded world. Technologically advanced modern hydro-infrastructure works wonders in affluent, highly regulated nations - think of how a vast arid region like Los Angeles has been transformed into a global megacity. It is, however, far less effective in coping with the technical inefficiencies and administrative ambiguity of fast-growing, less developed societies. For example, India - where it rains for four to six months each year - is facing the worst water crisis in its history. Per the government think tank NITI Aayog, an estimated 21 Indian cities have run out of groundwater by 2020. And even in cities that rely on industrial hydro-infrastructure for their water needs, there is a vast underserved demographic that has no access to such systems.

For us architects and urbanists, this gap underscores the relevance of vernacular infrastructure and pre-industrial indigenous systems that are an incredible yet underestimated part of our urban inheritance. Many such systems exist within and around our cities,

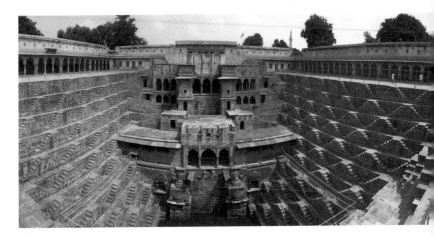

Figure 12.3
Chand Baori (stepped well), Rajasthan, India
Source: Gryffindor (see Image Credits for details)

often in neglected and abandoned conditions. Is the pandemic an opportunity for us to reflect deeper on their potential - beyond their historic value or their formal and aesthetic aspects? Can these systems be rethought as active infrastructural elements that can work in tandem with our modern infrastructure to bridge evident socio-economic gaps?

Consider for example the *hiti* water system of Nepal that has provided and distributed water for approximately 1,500 years. Upstream ponds or aquifers are connected to a depression in the ground through pipelines and canals, and eventually made visible as channelized spouts along a vertical wall, accompanied by tanks, wells, and even shrines, making them important religious settings. Today, Nepal's municipal systems are unable to provide adequate drinking water to residents due to limited infrastructural resources and weak management. In the Kathmandu Valley alone the low-income demographic depends on the 200-odd hiti systems still in working condition. As such, with the operation and maintenance

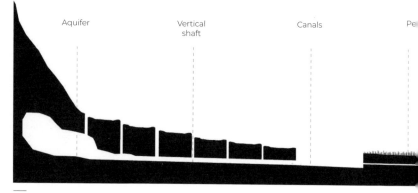

Mountain

Aquifer

Vertical shaft

Canals

Pe

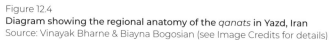

Figure 12.4
Diagram showing the regional anatomy of the *qanats* in Yazd, Iran
Source: Vinayak Bharne & Biayna Bogosian (see Image Credits for details)

of hitis already being part of local knowledge, their revitalization can make a significant and reliable contribution to the availability of fresh drinking water for a significant demographic in Nepal today.

Such indigenous systems have even greater relevance in areas of water scarcity. One thinks of the *qanats* - the historic subterranean water channels in the desert city of Yazd, Iran. The proximate Zagros Mountains gather snow in the winters forming a subterranean aquifer. Starting with a potential source-well, vertical shafts of successively increasing depths are dug at intervals and horizontally connected by subterranean sloped tunnels to enable water flow via gravity. Water from the mountain aquifer is guided into the peri-urban fields, and then into subterranean reservoirs, before directing it into individual pools within monuments and dwellings. The reservoirs called *ab anbars*, characterized by their large domes and cooling towers have also historically played a pivotal social role. Each ab anbar provided water to a limited number of streets and houses, defining a community shed around it and adding to the

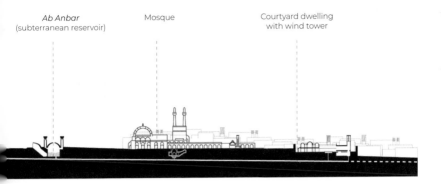

Ab Anbar
(subterranean reservoir)   Mosque   Courtyard dwelling
                                               with wind tower

formal structure of Yazd's historic neighborhoods as much as its mosques and madrassas.

Over the past six decades, these gravity-reliant systems have been unable to supply the vast amount of water needed for sprawling Iranian cities, and motorized wells and dams have subsequently gained dominance. Today, Yazd's principal water supply comes from modern pipelines from the Zayandehrud River more than 200 kilometers away. No new qanats have been constructed since 1963, and of the 3,300 within the Yazd Province, around 3,000 are increasingly polluted from industrial discharge. But qanats survive in Yazd's exurban agricultural fields, where their proximity to the mountains and source aquifer makes them economically and environmentally more efficient than wells.

Indigenous water systems have also generated magnificent landforms. For example, the Banaue Rice Terraces in the Cordillera Administrative Region of Luzon, Philippines. These colossal agricultural systems were carved into the mountains over centuries by the Ifugao people - largely by hand. They are composed of eight interrelated levels starting from public forests at the highest elevation, followed by privately owned forest lots, slash-and-burn farms, communal and cane grasslands, rice terraces, and, finally, the settlements and irrigation outflow rivers at the lowest level. Today these landscapes are threatened by contamination as well as economic pressures to maximize the rice production due to competition from industrial processes.

The polders of Bangladesh are another case in point. This network of coastal embankments consists of more than a million hectares of land at the cusp of three rivers - Ganga, Brahmaputra, and Meghna - intersected by numerous tributaries. They were constructed in the early 1960s to protect these low-lying areas from inundation and salinity intrusion with sluice gates allowing controlled water entry for agricultural production. Entire communities live within and around the network. And yet, since the beginning, they have been adversely impacted due to lack of maintenance, funding, and administration. From the *chinampas* (agrarian lake beds) of Mexico to the *baoris* (stepped wells) of India, numerous such examples of vernacular water-related urbanisms face an uncertain future.

As ingenious examples of harvesting, distributing, storing, and even celebrating water, the potential of these systems cannot be underestimated during this time. If given a place in our urbanization processes, whether in traditional or new forms, these systems can help cater to the needs of a significant urban demographic that urgently needs access to clean water. As our cities increase their sustainability prerogatives, these systems can inspire new planning directions with compact habitats sustained by local, decentralized, vernacular infrastructure rather than their industrial counterpart. And they can deepen our cultural understandings, because all such vernacular systems are inseparable from the cultural signatures of their place. The *madis* (water channels) of Isfahan, *tirthas* (sacred reservoirs) of Banaras, and fountains of Rome do not just supply water, they also contribute to the cultural identities of their respective locales.

The COVID-19 pandemic may well be a dress-rehearsal of the challenges of climate change and global warming that are lurking beyond. And while a vaccination may help take care of this pandemic, there certainly will not be one for climate change. Our professional efforts as architects and urbanists must therefore expand urgently to address these bigger concerns by collaborating with environmental, geographical, and social sciences. And this includes not just new development, but also the conservation of heritage habitats, infrastructures, and landscapes. The act of protecting, restoring, and reusing built elements of historic and cultural significance must be recognized as a far more reflective process of ecological and environmental reform.

While the pandemic has exacerbated the water crisis, it has also drawn our attention to it and highlighted why vernacular water urbanisms matter. In this regard, we architects and urbanists can expand ongoing dialogues to include these examples - not merely as architectural forms to emulate, but as didactic systems and places that can teach us about harmonious connections between ecology, sustainability, and habitat. We can critique the evident limitations of mainstream urbanization processes, and advocate for giving these systems a place in our city-making processes. Most importantly, we can help conserve, revive, and even reinvent these systems as parallel urban elements that can reach places and people in our cities where their modern counterparts cannot.

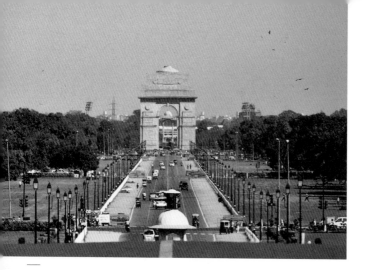

Figure 13.1
India Gate terminating Raj Path, New Delhi, India Source: Gughanbose
(see Image Credits for details)

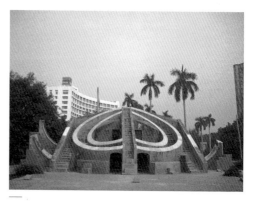

Figure 13.2
Jantar Mantar, New Delhi, India
Source: Abhijit Jawanjal (see Image Credits for
details)

13

Narratives of Protest

In any discussion on urbanism and the pandemic, one cannot afford to miss the numerous performances of protest. Amidst the COVID-19 lockdowns, these events seem like ostensible contradictions intent on revealing a darker hidden truth. In a time when we are confined to our dwellings due to the apparent risk to our own lives, the act of stepping out in droves to raise a voice against perceived injustice is far more than a mode of political expression. It is evidence that even something as seemingly daunting as a global pandemic can hardly interrupt people's ability to claim their cities in the wake of perceived institutional and administrative underperformance.

New Delhi, the capital of the world's most populous democracy, was one of the major global cities where mass protests were in full play just before the pandemic outbreak. On December 14, 2019, the Shaheen Bagh sit-in peaceful protest had begun in response to the passing of the Citizenship (Amendment) Act. Protestors continued to block a city road using non-violent resistance for 101 days, until March 24, 2020, when the Delhi Police vacated the site due to the pandemic.

In early March 2020, civil unrest broke throughout Chile in response to the increasing economic inequality in the country. On April 27, Lebanese citizens took to the streets to protest the nation's deteriorating economic situation. On May 26, tens of thousands of people in various cities across the United States protested the death of George Floyd. These protesters were not ignoring the pandemic. Most wore masks, some carried hand sanitizer, and others adhered to norms of physical distancing.

Performances of protest insinuate profound urban narratives. They offer important insights on the intersection of public space, contestation, and democracy. And sometimes, the choice of a protest site is in itself revealing. One recalls the famous Shinjuku Concerts in 1969 when 7,000 anti-Vietnam War activists crowded the subterranean spaces and passageways of Shinjuku Station to sing folk songs and listen to antiwar speeches. In an attempt to bring the people of Japan into contact with political activism, they excavated a new site for populist expression - a train station, not a plaza or park, became the new setting for performing the protest.

The encroachment on physical public spaces during such events is symbolic of the perceived encroachment made on the minds of people. Think of the "Free the Open Hand Campaign" in Chandigarh's Capitol Complex that led to making the Open Hand monument accessible to the public. On August 15 (India's Independence Day), 2010, scores of residents led by Hum Log (literally "We the People"), a local non-government organization, sang the national anthem at the Open Hand to mark the important day, and also highlight the Capitol's restricted access to the Chandigarh public. The administration had denied permission for this event citing security reasons, but the organizers filed a suit in the High Court obtaining permission to sing the anthem.

Cultures of protest impart their own identities on sites, monuments, and places, overlaying origins, authenticities, and histories, and imparting new meanings to them. Consider for instance Jantar Mantar, one of New Delhi's most recognizable monuments, an ensemble of astronomical instruments tracing back to the 18th century. Before the pandemic, the monument's identity was not dominated by the colorful historic science instruments, but riots of pamphlets and placards, dins of shouting slogans, droves of charged people in pitched tents peacefully protesting for all kinds of causes, and finally the uncanny entrepreneurship of snack kiosks and tea shops catering to these events each day.

Jantar Mantar was not the first choice as a place of protest in the city of New Delhi. Its predecessor was the Boat Club lawns - running along both sides of Rajpath, the original axial avenue of the colonial capital connecting India Gate to Rashtrapati Bhavan (the former Viceroy's Palace) up Raisana Hill. The shift occurred in October 1988, after Mahendra Singh Tikait led a protest with thousands of farmers from Uttar Pradesh along with their cattle, onto the lawns, lighting campfires and cooking food in the open for around a week. A consequent public interest litigation filed in the Supreme Court asked that the government find new places for protests in the city.

The focus shifted to Ramlila Maidan, the vast "pond" separating Old and New Delhi that was filled up in the early 1930s as the new site of the Ramlila Festival, and it quickly became a popular site for political events. It was here in June 1975 that Jayaprakash Narayan led his mammoth rally with over a lakh people protesting against Indira Gandhi's government. In 1977, following the emergency situation, several anti-Congress opposition leaders hosted a rally to form the Janata Party. And in August 2011, Anna Hazare performed his anti-corruption protest here.

In light of this pandemic and the health issues it surfaces, New Delhi's status as the world's most polluted capital city comes to the forefront. The city's air quality index (AQI) registers above 200 on a typical day and has even soared to a life-threatening 900 (anything above 25 is labelled unsafe by World Health Organization). Since the lockdowns, before and after photographs of another colonial monument in the city, India Gate, have been gaining attention. The visual contrast of the massive gate seen with and without the city's polluted air is striking. This 43-meter-high monument located on the eastern edge of the city's ceremonial axis was originally built to pay tribute to the 70,000 soldiers of the British Indian Army who had died in the First World War. Since 1971, it has served as India's tomb of the unknown soldier. In November 2019, more than 1,500 people gathered here protesting the city's alarmingly high pollution levels and demanding action from the federal and state governments.

Less than six months since the protest, and three weeks since India's COVID-19 lockdown on March 24, 2020, 11 million vehicles were taken off from New Delhi's roads, while factories and construction came to a halt. For the first time in the city's recent history, air pollution dropped below 20. The skies appeared blue during the day, and starry at night. The November protest witnessed a welcome result through government action, even though it was not a response to the protest. It is just that the pandemic had a silver lining to it.

Even as the pandemic puts a pause on traditional forms of protest, millions of people, from Delhi to Chile to the United States, have been voicing their discontent through alternative and adapted means. While these events may embody numerous urban emotions - from patriotism and peace to desperate cries against social and economic injustice - they also represent the difficult ways in which people are compelled to communicate their loss. As forms of publicness, such events are therefore evidence of the conflict between people's aspirations and a less sanitized display of a city's reality. They underscore the idea of public space as the contested and negotiated terrain of socio-political renewal. They affirm the rights of citizens to gauge the effectiveness of their governments. And they offer us profound lenses - such as representation, participation, transparency, accountability, equality - to re-read our cities as evolving dialectics of democracy, and by extension to re-read democracy as a culturally filtered phenomenon.

Performances of protest remind us that while our cities may be designed, built, and experienced as three-dimensional physical places, they are in fact phenomena in flux, events in time. Recognizable places and monuments in our cities are never at rest. Numerous unwitting events expand their originating histories, skew their identities, and even transform their legacies in ways no one can predict - at once an architectural and anthropological riddle. The most identifiable destinations in our cities must therefore never be understood through narrow and exclusively historic or nostalgic mind-frames. Within and around their shifting identities are far deeper revelations of our socio-political cleavages and scars, and the simultaneous re-appraisal of our collective societal aspirations.

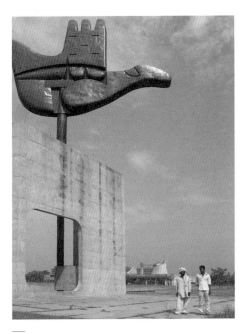

Figure 13.3
Open Hand monument, Chandigarh, India
Source: Author

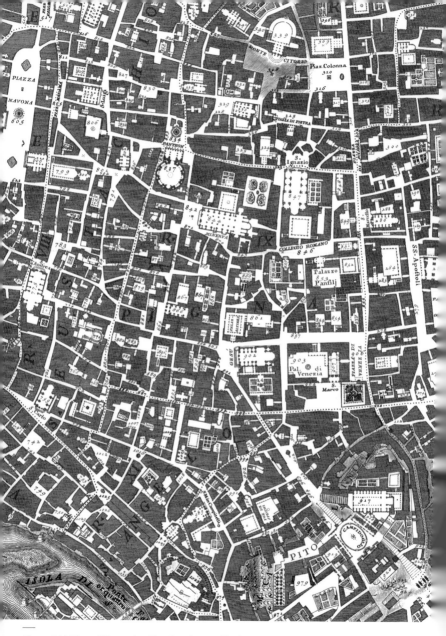

Figure 14.1 **Plan of Rome by Giambattista Nolli, circa 1748.** Source: Public Domain

14

The Arts and the City

Some of us think of the arts as frivolous, self-indulgent endeavors, but the fact is that they play a consequential role in defining the everyday well-being our societies, particularly in hard times - such as this pandemic. Beyond their cultural value, they are instruments of communication and identity. They strengthen communal bonds, blur social differences, and bridge economic gaps. They reinforce inclusiveness and heritage identity. They raise awareness and inspire action on pressing issues such as environmental degradation and climate change, validating their deeper purpose in urban advocacy and activism.

There has always been a profound relationship between the arts and cities, and the urban landscape has, throughout human history, captured the attention of the most gifted artistic minds. The meticulous 11th-century, five-meter-long painting Qingming Shanghe Tu depicts daily life in Song Dynasty China. Giovanni Battista Piranesi's 220 engravings (1756) record the vanishing past of the Roman Empire. The woodcut prints of Utagawa Hiroshige titled Fifty-Three Stations of the Tokaido (1832) capture scenes along the road connecting Tokyo and Kyoto. And the sketches of British urbanist Gordon Cullen from his seminal 1961 book, Townscape, analyze the city as a sequential visual composition. The artistic representations of our cities are a means to celebrate our relationship with them.

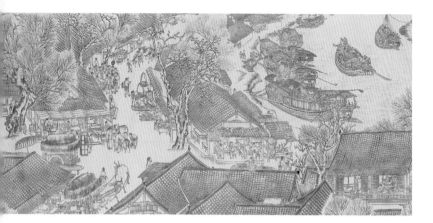

Figure 14.2
A small section of the Qingming Shanghe Tu, the 11th-century, five-meter-long painting, by Zhang Zeduan (1085–1145) depicting daily life in Song Dynasty China
Source: Public Domain

But how we choose to represent a city is also evidence of how we choose to see it. For example, the 1748 mapping of Renaissance Rome by the architect/surveyor Giambattista Nolli meticulously documents the form of the city's public spaces both within and outside buildings. Yet, it is inept in depicting undulating terrains, making Rome appear flat. It reduces Rome's layered history to a singular dimension of black and white, and says nothing about how people actually experience public space. Rome, in the Nolli Plan, is an "empty city," just like our cities have been during the lockdowns. By contrast, the 18th-century Japanese painted screens called Ryakuchu Ryakugai Zu depict the Kyoto cityscape as a dynamic setting of people, seasons, rituals, and festivals shrouded in golden clouds. They prioritize activity over urban form. Both contrasting representations have deep relevance to our understanding of cities. But taken in isolation, they remain incomplete due to their specific biases.

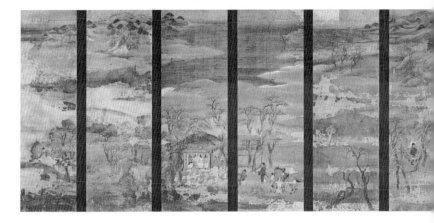

Figure 14.3
A section of an 11th - 12th century six-panel silk screen, Kyoto, Japan
Source: Public Domain

There are of course myriad other arts through which we explore the urban. Charles Dickens's (1812–1870) long walks in the streets of Victorian London inspired his literary descriptions of the sights, sounds, and smells of the city. Hope Mirrlees's Paris: A Poem (1919) narrates her daylong stroll from metro tunnels and city streets to gardens and museums. Charlie Chaplin's 1931 film City Lights explores themes of migration, homelessness, and the search for a place in the urban milieu. And Ridley Scott's 1982 science-fiction noir Blade Runner is unthinkable without its backdrop of a dreary, dark Los Angeles lost to industrial blight.

The city also emanates the maverick artist within us. On the one hand, graffiti, as a rebellious art created without permission, is seen by civic authorities as a form of vandalism. On the other, popu-list art and craft created during festive events are testimony to a city's unspoken tolerance and order: The artistic transformation of

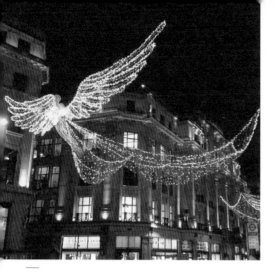

Figure 14.4
Christmas decorations in Regent Street, London, United Kingdom, in 2017. Source: Simeon87 (see Image Credits for details)

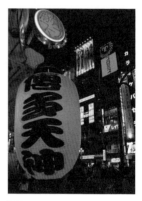

Figure 14.5
Traditional paper lantern, Tokyo, Japan
Source: Author

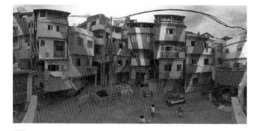

Figure 14.6
Santa Marta favela painting by Haas & Hahn
Source: André Sampaio (see Image Credits for details)

Mumbai's districts with lights, fetishes, and paper lanterns during Diwali, or the luminous Christmas nightscape of London's Regent Street are evidence of our collective urge to aestheticize our cities as expressions of communal and civic celebration.

The most profound relationship that the arts share with the city is through their transformative potential to reinforce civic pride and catalyze positive socio-cultural change. In 2010, Dutch artists Haas & Hahn returned to the Santa Marta favela in Rio de Janeiro, Brazil, to paint over 34 houses, covering an area of 7,000 square meters. The objective was to create community art at a big scale to serve as a catalyst for improving the housing conditions within the neighborhoods. By empowering the people and bringing color and joy into their unplanned environment, Haas & Hahn ignited personal and societal change on all levels. It brought smiles on the faces of slum dwellers just like the Ouzville art project did in Lebanon seven years later. Here, a former resident of this evaded neighborhood invited artists to paint giant murals on neglected buildings, while gathering volunteers to clean the streets of garbage.

While all such efforts were brought to an abrupt halt by lockdowns across the world, cities and countries are gradually easing stay-at-home restrictions, and numerous artists are once again engaging with the city. Far from being absent, street art is in fact deriving inspiration from the pandemic. It is offering comic relief, wit, and beauty and sending messages of hope and despair in a time when we are all separated from each other. In Los Angeles, local artist Ponywave has captured love during the pandemic in a street mural showing two people kissing while wearing masks. In Berlin, Gollum from Lord of the Rings utters his signature words, "My Precious," while looking ardently at a roll of toilet paper. In Jaipur, graffiti on an empty road shows a green coronavirus with a dangling red tongue saying "Stay Home, Save Lives." And in Amsterdam, a mural by the artist FAKE shows a female health-care worker in a face mask with the Supergirl symbol.

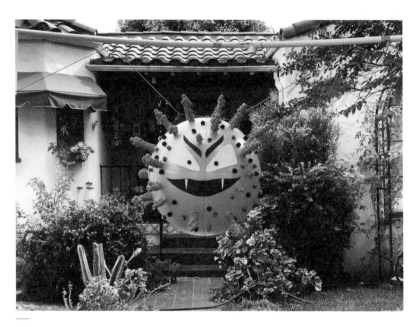

Figure 14.7
"Coronavirus" art installation in a front yard in Pasadena, California, during Halloween 2020. Source: Author

In the United States, the City of Boulder's Office of Arts and Culture has partnered with Create Boulder, a network of local leaders, to launch "Creative Neighborhood: COVID-19 Work Projects." The program delivers funding to artists who have lost work due to pandemic-related restrictions leveraging their talents to enhance community bonds. For example, the Avant Gardens project invites community members to create do-it-yourself botanical sculptures with living plants and found objects as memorials for those affected by the pandemic. In another project, a vocalist performs for the neighborhood from his backyard, and neighbors in adjacent yards sing along and make requests. Sixty-six projects - ranging from music and theater to visual art and art education - are currently underway in various parts of the city.

On May 29, 2020, the New Zealand government announced a $175 million relief package to boost the creative sector in the wake of the pandemic. It concluded that this sector, without government intervention, would be hit twice as hard as the rest of the country's economy, and the initiative is expected to help up to 2,000 jobs in the creative industry over the next four years. One could argue that such initiatives are easier done in small, affluent societies such as New Zealand with a limited population of merely 4.9 million - the size of a modest city in other parts of the world. Which is precisely why cities could serve to learn a lot from this. Particularly when one appreciates New Zealand's ranking in seventh place (the first six countries being from Europe) in the annual Legatum Prosperity Index - which is not just based on wealth and economic growth, but other aspects such as education, health, personal well-being, and quality of life.

In a time when the very concept of urban space and public life is being challenged, the arts are helping us reclaim the everyday city to express our collective anguish. They are debunking the assumption that we indulge in the artistic only when our basic aspects are satisfied. Art is a fundamental human need, and the city is the largest canvas one can hope for. As we wait impatiently for the pandemic to pass, we must not fail to notice the global "COVID-19 art gallery" emerging all around us. It is letting us speak to each other across boundaries and borders. It is enabling us to hear each other amidst our increasing privatization. It is bringing smiles to millions of faces in these difficult times.

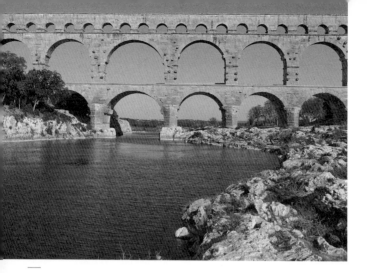

Figure 15.1 **The Pont du Gard, an ancient Roman aqueduct bridge built the first century CE, carried water over 50 kilometers**
Source: Roberto Ferrari (see Image Credits for details)

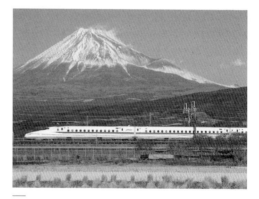

Figure 15.2
An N700 series Shinkansen bullet train in Japan, with Mount Fuji in the background.
Source: Tansaisuketti (see Image Credits for details)

15

Technology and the City

We live in a time when technology has broken physical and territorial barriers. Think of the unprecedented speed at which not just information, but people and goods move across the world today. Back in 1499, it took Portuguese explorers more than half a year to discover Goa by ship. It would take them merely 10 hours to get there today by plane. Yet this very pace of geographic locomotion has spread the virus across oceans, generating the global pandemic.

The ever-increasing velocity of transportation and capital has even transformed something as fundamental as food. For example, the Tsukiji Market in Tokyo, from where thousands of tons of seafood were frozen, cut, packed, and flown to every corner of the world, was the heart of a global phenomenon called sushi. The Toyosu fish market, which opened in 2018 to replace it, is subsequently facing a difficult time during the pandemic with collapsed fish trade and global demand.

The astounding speed of building construction during this pandemic is a reminder of how far we have come as city builders. In Wuhan, China, the construction of the 1,000-patient Caidian Huoshenshan Hospital was started on January 23, 2020 and it was put into operation only a few days later on February 2. It was completed by four contractor teams and built in this short time frame because of its modular structure. On February 3, three other hospitals began construction in the city - at the Wuhan Hongshan Stadium, Wuhan Salon, and Wuhan International Convention and Exhibition Center, and the following day, it was announced that the surrounding areas would build eight additional temporary hospitals to treat COVID-19 patients.

Digital media has come into a new light during the pandemic, particularly due to the need for effective data gathering for public-health purposes. For example, "Worldometer" is a reference website that provides real-time statistics on diverse topics - including the number of people across the world known to have COVID-19. WhatsApp has partnered with the Singapore government to provide the public daily updates about COVID-19 cases. But simultaneously, the impact of misinformation during an outbreak also cannot be undermined. As noted in the World Health Organization Situation Report 13, the COVID-19 pandemic bears the danger of being accompanied by a massive "infodemic" - an "over-abundance of information - some accurate and some not - that makes it hard for people to find trustworthy sources." How did we get to this point where "invisible technology" is not just shaping local institutions but influencing global processes and perceptions?

In the past, the most ambitious projects were related to something as fundamental as water - one thinks of Rome's ancient aqueducts such as the Aqua Appia (315 BCE) that ran for 16.4 kilometers and dropped 10 meters to discharge 73,000 cubic meters of water into the city each day. The advanced naval technology of the European powers and their possession of a Chinese Tang dynasty (9th century CE) invention called gunpowder led to the entire history of colonization. Water was a more efficient means of transportation than roads, and this led to massive regional infrastructure projects - the 193-kilometer-long Suez Canal joining the Mediterranean and Red Seas in 1856, and the 82-kilometer-long Panama Canal joining the Pacific and Atlantic Oceans in 1914.

A paradigmatic shift in urban form occurred through three techno-logical advances: the steam-powered factory, the railroad transpor-tation system, and the commercial production of the automobile. In the United States, the 1956 Federal Aid Highway Act authorized the construction of 66,000 kilometers of the highways over a 10-year period. In Los Angeles, which boasted one of the most extensive train networks in the world, 1,600 kilometers of rail were disman-tled and by 1963 overlaid by an extensive freeway system. The auto-mobile now connected a central business district to proliferating single-family suburbs that ate up the countryside. Three decades after the inauguration of one of the nation's first freeways in 1940, the words "smog," "gridlock," and "sprawl" were being increasingly uttered in several cities in North America.

Meanwhile, in Manhattan, New York, the Chrysler Building - an Art Deco skyscraper - stood at 1,046 feet as the world's tallest building for 11 months before it was surpassed by the Empire State Building in 1931. And while the city soared toward the sky, it also burrowed into the ground. In less than four decades, by the 1970s, a vast subterranean network of shopping tunnels, retail nodes, and transit stations was emerging as a parallel urban world in large cities such as Toronto and Tokyo.

Our cities changed again at the dawn of the 21st century through globalization and the evolution of information technology - the first commercial installation of the fiber-optic cable in 1977; the first IBM PC hitting the markets in 1981; the first version of the Windows operating system being shipped in 1985; and the founding of the money transfer system PayPal in 1998. As Thomas Friedman noted in his 2005 Pulitzer Prize-winning book, The World Is Flat, just like the freeways in the fifties had "flattened" the United States, easing the movement of people and goods, so had "the laying of global fiber highways flattened the developed world." What the car wash was to the Machine Age, the internet café is to this new era of easy travel, social media, globalized banking, and the worldwide web.

But in a time when more than 600 million people across the world live on less than US $1.90 a day, and when, per World Bank data, the pandemic is expected to increase global extreme poverty in 2020 for the first time in over two decades, the urgent question at hand is how to expand the positive impacts of technology to all. The increasing reliance on digital technology during the lockdowns, for example, has highlighted this issue in less affluent nations. For example, the July 2017–June 2018 report of the National Statistical Office of the Government of India showed that only 24% of Indian households have internet access, and only 11% of households possess any type of computer. In places like India, online classrooms therefore do not translate into effective remote learning; in fact they enlarge the inequity gap in educational outcomes, distancing the underprivileged to the fringes of the education system. As Protiva Kundu from the Centre for Budget and Governance Accountability notes, the COVID-19 pandemic has thus "exposed how rooted structural imbalances are between rural and urban, male and female, rich and poor, even in the digital world."

Bridging these gaps remains a challenge but there are worthy ongoing efforts in this regard. Loon LLC, for example, is an Alphabet Inc. subsidiary working to provide internet access to rural and remote areas. It uses balloons at an altitude of 18–25 kilometers to create an aerial wireless network. The balloons are maneuvered using wind data from the National Oceanic and Atmospheric Administration (NOAA). Users connect to the network using a special internet antenna attached to their building. The signal travels from balloon to balloon, and eventually to an on-ground station connected to an internet service provider. A recent blog by Salvatore Candido, a Loon LLC Chief Technology Officer, claimed a record-duration flight of 312 days for a balloon that was launched from Puerto Rico in May 2019 and landed in Baja, Mexico in March 2020.

Along with such innovative ideas, the strategic amalgamation of technical and human resources is of crucial importance in less developed societies. Take the case of something as simple as a mobile phone. David Edelstein, who co-leads Grameen Foundation's global programs, explains how in Uganda, Community Knowledge Workers equipped with cell phones spend a portion of the day visiting local farmers, learning about crop diseases, market prices, and how to maximize yields - thereby helping the farming community increase productivity by sharing much-needed information. According to a 2012 World Bank report, more than 2.5 billion people across the world without access to a bank account are now using mobile phone services to collect payments and transfer money. International non-government organizations such as Malaria No More are using mobile technology to combat diseases, with diagnostic tests, reliable drugs, and even bed nets made available through SMS mobile phone campaigns.

The pandemic is reminding us that the impact of science and technology only goes as far as its ability to be accessible to all. This is where our leaders and administrators have a crucial role to play - to ensure than no one in our cities will be left out. In a time when easy global travel has direct impacts on this outbreak, our radius of concern must expand far beyond our local, regional, and national boundaries. The pandemic is an instance where the health of one society cannot afford to come at the expense of another. The pandemic is revealing a far deeper truth: that we live in an interdependent, interconnected world. Technology may be a means to a better future, but it is certainly not the only one. Our health, habits, choices, attitudes, and spheres of concern are of even greater importance in this regard. The pandemic is testing our technological limits. More importantly, it is reminding us of the limits of technology.

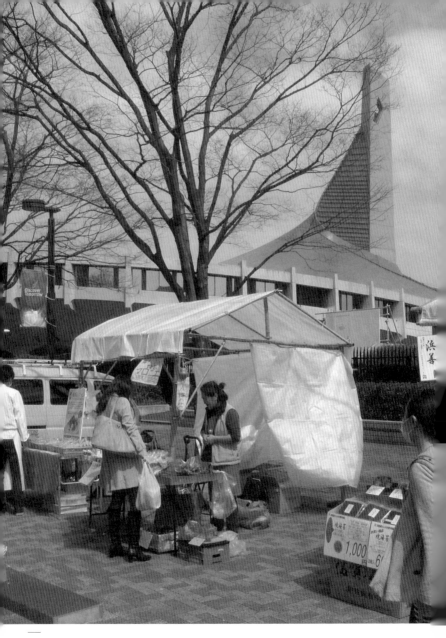

Figure 16.1 **Farmers market in front of Yoyogi stadium, Tokyo, Japan.** Source: Author

16

The Edited City

Barren and desolate photographs of Saint Marks Piazza in Venice, Capitoline Hill in Rome, or Taj Mahal in Agra, during the lockdowns are affirmations of the degree to which tourism, travel, and recreational activity has come to an abrupt standstill during this unprecedented time. It is as if someone has edited these photographs using computer software. As if someone in a whiff of jest has erased all humans to assert a perverse point. The empty COVID-19 non-human city is surreal, even apocalyptic.

But aren't such photos without people exactly the kind that we architects love taking; the kind that inundate architecture volumes and magazines? Some years back I was in Tokyo, walking uphill with a well-known architect friend from Shibuya Station to the Meiji Shrine. We passed by a farmers market in front of the Yoyogi Stadium, designed by the famous Japanese architect Kenzo Tange in the late 1950s. My friend pulled out his camera in excitement. Then he complained that he could not get a clean shot of the famous building, because the tents and people were interrupting his frame. I was amazed at his reaction. I found the market in front of the building far more interesting than the bare photos of the sculptural stadium I had seen in books as an architecture student. When I look back, none of those photographs had any people in them. They had been edited to highlight only the clarity of the architectural form.

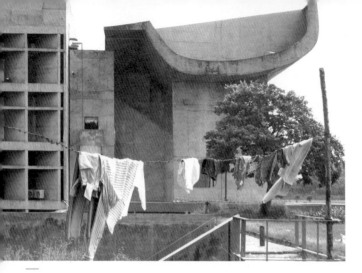

Figure 16.2
Clothes hung to dry in front of the Assembly Complex, Chandigarh, India
Source: Author

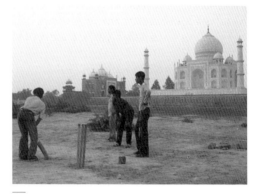

Figure 16.3
Villagers appropriate the dried Yamuna riverbed as a cricket field in front of Taj Mahal, Agra, India
Source: Author

I can recall a similar experience the first time I visited the Capitol Complex in Chandigarh - designed by Le Corbusier in the 1950s. Since my student days, I had admired the sheer chutzpah of this vast brutal landscape against the Himalayan backdrop, and the sculptural formalism of the Assembly, High Court, and Secretariat. But the Capitol I saw in 2010 had guard posts, gates, and barbed wire fences interrupting my view of the buildings. Weeds occupied the vast concrete esplanade between them. The Open Hand monument and as its sunken plaza conceived for public debate appeared forlorn and brooding. Circa 1985, some three decades after the Capitol's opening, Chandigarh had been gripped by the paranoia of Sikh terrorists killing people at will. Emergency security measures were implemented to safeguard the administrative center fortifying the entire precinct.

What surprised me was that the Capitol had never been presented this way in succeeding architecture and planning volumes. It had been projected only as an original Corbusian figment. Its photographs were either from the early fifties, before any of this had happened, or they had been carefully edited to erase the barbed wires, gateposts, and weeds, and showcase only the sculptural buildings. The books had always celebrated the Chandigarh Capitol as Le Corbusier's achievement, and the only thing that mattered was his original vision, not its legacy. As a student, I had been duped into seeing the Capitol through a manipulated viewpoint that had disconnected its history and denied me any knowledge of its evolving identity.

I can say the same for Taj Mahal. In September 2010, the Yamuna River touched the base of the Taj Mahal's 300-meter-long river-facing terrace for the first time in more than two decades. Heavy rains in north India had raised the river's water level creating a momentous event in the recent history of the monument that had fronted a near-dry riverbed for too long. This event forced tourists, who are hardly aware of the river's presence, to notice it. Most entering through the magnificent red sandstone gateway are euphoric to see the Taj Mahal's dominant media image - a frontal white building with four minars and a quadrangular garden. Many climb up the mausoleum's base, some go behind the building and discover the river for the first time, but few understand its significance to the monument's design. Several studies have now concluded that the strength of the wooden shafts holding together Taj Mahal's foundation depends on being constantly moistened by the river's water.

This is only half of the Taj Mahal story. The other half remains shrouded within Taj Gunj - the informal habitat directly south of it. This is, in fact, the former *caravanserai* (commercial precinct) of the Taj Mahal's 22-hectare campus, that in the mid-seventeenth century was teeming with local and foreign trade. Consequent to the Mughal capital's shift to Delhi, the market declined, and was incrementally appropriated by local merchants to meet their growing demands. By the early 20th century its four quads had been filled in with haphazard development, reducing the streets to tenuous lanes. Today, there is little to reveal the caravanserai's original form as one steps out of the mausoleum garden into the court that was once the transition between the two. And with the tourist entry located at the court's eastern approach, one is made to turn northward to enter the mausoleum precinct bypassing the door that leads to the Gunj. For most, the experience of the Taj Mahal begins and ends with a white building and its immediate garden.

How easily we weed out the so called "dirty," "ordinary" world that surrounds our architectural landmarks. How conveniently we "edit" the evolving history of a place and erase urban realities through the filter of our self-imposed biases. Why are origins the only ways through which we choose to see our buildings? Why can't other dimensions - like appropriation, possession, transformation - be accepted and celebrated as intrinsic parts of a building's evolving history, or even its irrevocable destiny?

I remember reading about the eminent American architect Robert Venturi's first trip to Japan, which came very late in his career in

1990. Having never been there, his impressions of Japan had been shaped by those of his Modern architect peers. But what Venturi saw in Japan with his own eyes shocked him. He realized that his predecessors had missed the point. Due to their modernist preoccupations, they had limited their perceptions to the sublime austerity and structural clarity of traditional Japanese buildings. They had chosen to ignore the vivid hues of moving kimonos, and the myriad colors of the Japanese seasons, wayside markets and commercial signs. Venturi returned home with numerous little objects from Japan's streets and flea markets - dolls, chopsticks, and idols made of paper, bamboo, and lacquered wood - and displayed them at the Philadelphia Museum of Art in 1995 under the title "Skill, Care, and Wit: Miscellaneous Objects from Japanese Markets."

How wonderful (and humbling) would it be if architects were to see their buildings not merely as sculptural objects, but evolving entities that are maturing through unpredictable, unforeseen forces far beyond the original ones that shaped them. This is the contrast between a self-referential architecture that denies its surrounds versus one that embraces it. This is the difference between looking at buildings in isolation versus reading them as components of the larger places within which they are situated. This difference is of crucial importance because how we read a place determines how we engage with it.

The photographs of famous buildings devoid of everyday life that we see during this pandemic are neither edited, nor manicured. They are as real as can be. Uncomfortable as they seem, they may serve well to remind architects to relax our aesthetic and formal obsessions with the buildings we create and embrace the truisms of spontaneous urban activity. An iconic building without the everyday reality that surrounds it is as unnatural as the empty cities we are experiencing during the COVID-19 lockdowns.

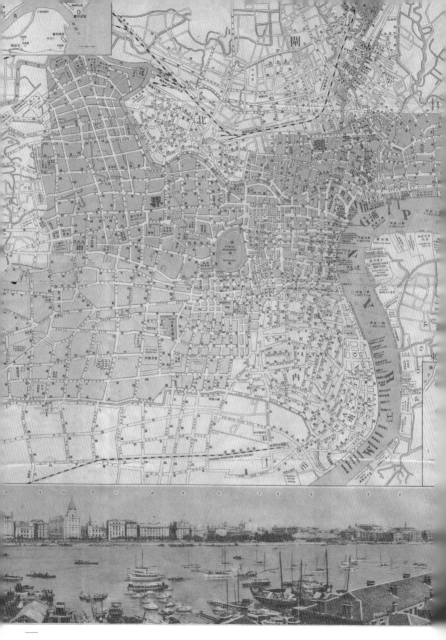

Figure 17.1 **A portion of the circa 1937 map of Shanghai, with a panoramic photo of the Bund along the bottom.** Source: Public Domain

17

A View from the Shanghai Bund

For the 24 million residents of Shanghai, the most populous city in the world's most populous nation, the 2020 Chinese New Year will remain etched in memory. Following the COVID-19 outbreak, on January 23, 2020, two days before the Chinese New Year, a full lockdown was announced in Wuhan, situated merely four hours by train from Shanghai. Hours later, the residents of Shanghai too found themselves trapped in their apartments.

With Shanghai in lockdown, the magnificent 1.5-kilometer-long Bund along the western waterfront of the Huangpu River that was supposed to be flooded with millions of revelers appeared like a ghost town. The term *bund* originates from a Persian word meaning embankment, levee, or dam. But the Chinese name for the Bund - *wai tan* - literally translates as "outer beach," because of its location downstream from the "inner" area adjacent to Shanghai's older walled city. It begins at Yan'an Road in the south and ends at Waibaidu Bridge in the north, crossing the Suzhou Creek.

During the lockdown, in the absence of people and activity, the contrast between Puxi's (the river's western bank) and Pudong's (the river's eastern bank) architecture and built fabric must have appeared even more vivid. Puxi's ensemble of hierarchical streets, pedestrian-scaled blocks, and street-friendly stone-, and brick-clad mid-rise build-

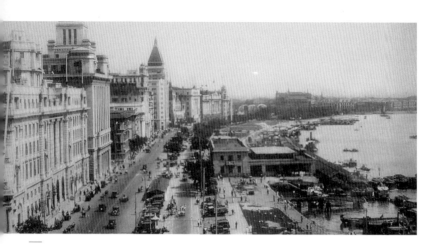

Figure 17.2
Colonial buildings along the Bund in Puxi (the river's western bank), circa 1930.
Source: Public Domain

ings is an incredible repository of the city's colonial history. In direct contrast, Pudong's skyline, in its high-rise scale, form, glass, and steel is an emblem of China's proclamation to the global stage. Puxi and Pudong, as contrasting identities, represent two chapters that narrate the story of Shanghai's evolution at a high decibel level.

The Bund centers on a section of Zhongshan Road in what was formerly the Shanghai International Settlement originating from the 1863 merger of the British and American enclaves. Shanghai's colonization traces back to June 1832 when a crew of about 70 individuals led by Hugh Hamilton Lindsay under the employment of the East India Company docked in the port of Shanghai for 18 days. Noticing more than five million tons of cargo being transported via this port, he began to realize its strategic importance second only to Guangzhou. The ensuing military conflict, famously known as the Opium War, led to the defeat of the Qing Dynasty government and the signing of the Treaty of Nanking with Britain on August 28, 1842.

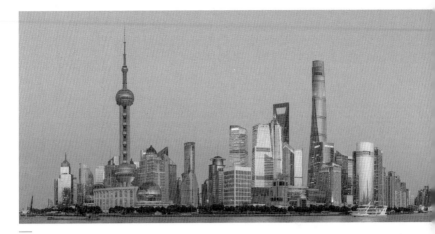

Figure 17.3
The glitzy skyline of Pudong (the river's eastern bank)
Source: Public Domain

The colonial buildings in Puxi – more than 50 of them in various architectural styles from Romanesque Revival, Gothic Revival, Renaissance Revival, and Baroque Revival, to Neo-Classical and Art Deco - are emblematic of this era. Many of them sprang up around the turn of the 20th century as the Bund began to develop into a major financial center in east Asia with banks and trading houses from the United Kingdom, France, the United States, and Russia. Today, within this protected historic district, one finds the wit and spontaneity of every urban life and appropriation - drying clothes, bicycles, fruit stalls, and snack shops all seamlessly juxtaposed against a robust concrete and stone architecture of permanence and impeccable detail.

One also sees this rich urban life in Shanghai's colonial neighborhoods like the ones built by the French Concession. It was established on April 6, 1849, after the French Consul to Shanghai, Charles de Montigny, obtained permission to build a settlement. Here,

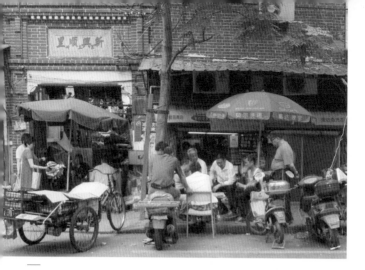

Figure 17.4
Street life in the French Concession neighborhood in Shanghai
Source: Author

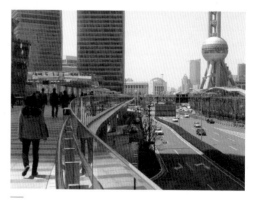

Figure 17.5
Skybridge in Pudong
Source: Author

numerous *linong* (two-story residential blocks) have arrays of north- and south-facing residential units with gated walls connecting their shorter sides to make a continuous street wall. In such neighborhoods, streets teeming with local retail are the armature of communal life, going from massive boulevards at the neighborhood edge to intimate arterials with trees fully covering the right-of way.

This harmony of Puxi's historic colonial district is literally the opposite of what one sees in Pudong's glitzy skyline. Pudong includes the Luijiazui Financial District, the Waigaoqiao Free Trade Zone, the Zhangjiang Hi-tech Park for technology-oriented businesses, and the industrial area of the Jinqiao Export Processing Zone. These areas have special perks such as lower export taxes employed through free-market principles, and due to its size and importance as China's financial hub, Pudong in fact has the equivalent status of a sub-provincial city.

But Pudong is not really a city. It is a collage of commercial districts, with some expensive and dramatic architecture including the 93-story, 420-meter-high Jin Mao Tower, the 101-story, 493-meter-high Shanghai World Financial Center, and the 468-meter-high Oriental Pearl Radio & Television Tower. Each of Pudong's skyscrapers stand as freestanding objects with wide swaths of asphalt separating them. Luijiazui's eight-lane Century Boulevard has four bicycle lanes and two pavements as wide as the traffic lanes. Unlike Puxi, there is no street-level retail, and shopping is confined to luxury indoor malls entered via sky bridges from the subway station. With a growing middle-class and a 70-billion-dollar GDP, this vibrant built-from-scratch financial district is the city's most ambitious statement of its rapid expansion over the past two decades.

It is hard to believe that Pudong's 1,200-odd square kilometer Special Economic Zone was largely agrarian villages as late as 1993. In barely 10 years it transformed into a five-million-inhabitant urbanity - something quite unthinkable by conventional Western standards. Until about 1984, the core of Shanghai's 308-square-kilometer urban area was centered on Puxi. Within as less as two decades, the number increased to more than 1,300 square kilometers. While the core radiated outward to include several exurban towns, the rural district east of Huangpu River became the site for constructing some of Shanghai's most iconic buildings. Per a 2015 World Bank report, more than 7,000 square kilometers (an area equivalent to 88 Manhattans) in the Yangtze River Delta Economic Zone - which includes Shanghai, Suzhou, Wuxi, and several other cities - became urbanized between 2000 and 2010.

In such a rapidly developing mega-city, the price to conserve a historic skyline such as Puxi's is high. The skyscrapers that have emerged on the blocks just behind the Bund's protected buildings are evidence of this development pressure. Which is why the care and attention to conserving Puxi's colonial district, and by extension, other colonial areas within the city, should and can be an inspiring lesson for several other fast-growing cities across Asia. It speaks volumes on how Shanghai sees its heritage buildings as cultural assets and built resources whose conservation plays a significant role in the urban economy. It suggests that in as much as Shanghai seeks to express its global aspirations through the innovative modern skyline of Pudong, it has simultaneously embraced the idea that its historic architecture bears its own value.

Over the past 25 years, the Bund's historic architectural waterfront has been through several conservation efforts. In 1996, the first conservation project cleaned up more than 100,000 square meters of the exterior walls of historic buildings. Beginning with the former HSBC Building (now housing the Shanghai Pudong Development Bank), numerous interior and exterior renovations followed, all maintaining the historic facades and architectural styles.

Other efforts included an extensive listing of historic buildings, streets and areas to be conserved throughout the city. Detailed definitions for building and open space conservation were accompanied by progressive urban design legislation and planning to ensure that setbacks and building profiles in new developments would be compatible with their historic counterparts. 41 areas including the Bund, and the Hengshan-Fuxing historic areas (a former French Concession), and more than 144 historic streets, such as Fuxing Road are part of this list. This is not something too many Asian cities can boast of, at least not at this scale.

Since April 6, 2020, following the relaxation of the lockdown rules, ambitious projects have been initiated in Shanghai to trigger an economic rebound. They include transforming 3.3 square kilometers of the riverside just north of the Bund into 8.4-million square meters of new development. An estimated 70,000 people will reside and 240,000 more will work in this new North Bund.

As the Bund awaits its new identity, the contrasting images of Puxi and Pudong are reminders that great cities are complex collages of layers of history, multiple utopias, and simultaneous initiatives of conservation and innovation. Cities evolve, times change, and emerging built forms continue to embody the evolving aspirations and ambitions of their times. For all the opinions we may have of what is right and wrong, the two urbanisms along the Huangpu River, in their presence and unapologetic contrast, will continue to make the Shanghai Bund one of the most unique and spectacular places in the world.

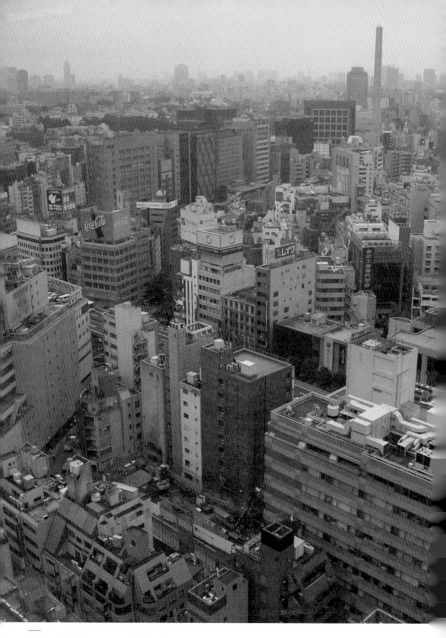

Figure 18.1 **Cityscape of Tokyo, Japan**
Source: Michael Greenhalgh (see Image Credits for details)

18

Embracing Uncertainty

I am reflecting today on urbanism and uncertainty, not because we are riding through a pandemic, but because some hundred major fires have burned across the West Coast of the United States this year in 2020. On August 16 and 17, thunderstorms in northern California came with more than 10,000 lightning strikes sparking more than 300 fires within 72 hours, and they have charred more than 350,000 acres, making this fire season one of the most active in the state's history. In Oregon, more than half-million people have had to flee their homes with mass evacuations underway across the region. The fires are not just overwhelming fire-fighters but also polluting the air from Los Angeles to Seattle. Officials are urging people to stay indoors, not due to the pandemic but bad air quality. Amidst what appears like an apocalyptic movie scene, a vibe of uncertainty looms all around us.

As a Los Angeles resident, I am reminded today of Mike Davis's 1999 book Ecology of Fear: Los Angeles and the Imagination of Disaster. He had argued that Southern California has reaped flood, fire, and earthquake tragedies that were potentially avoidable because "for generations, market-driven urbanization has transgressed environmental common sense," and because "historic wildfire corridors have been turned into view-lot suburbs, wetland liquefaction zones into marinas, and flood plains into indus-

A. Circa 1630.
Edo Era

B. Circa 1657.
City destroyed
by the Great
Meireki Fire

C. Circa 1670.
Tokyo rebuilt

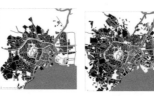

D. Circa 1868.
Tokyo grows in
the Meiji and
Taisho Era

E. Circa 1923.
Tokyo destroyed
by the Great Kanto
Earthquake

F. Circa 1940.
Tokyo rebuilt

G. Circa 1945.
Tokyo destroyed
by bombing in the
Second World War

H. Circa 2020.
Tokyo today

Figure 18.2
Evolution of Tokyo
Source: Author

trial districts and housing tracts." To think that Los Angeles, one of the great mega-cities on the planet is situated on a vulnerable geology susceptible to natural hazards seems counter-intuitive. There are over a hundred small active faults in the region that can cause damaging earthquakes like the Northridge earthquake in 1994. Wildfire and drought dominate the state's climate change debates even as the sea level around San Francisco has risen by six inches since 1950.

And so, in my anxious state, I look to Tokyo today, another mega-city located in a disaster-prone natural geography. The Japanese archipelago sits at the nexus of four tectonic plates, subjecting the region to more than 1,500 annual seismic events, including at least two 5.0 magnitude or higher earthquakes. Tokyo, with over nine million occupants, is situated on one of its most fragile geologies. Los Angeles's vast horizontal explosion and Tokyo's land-pressure driven implosion could not be more different, but I can appreciate all the more today what I have observed and learnt from my visits to Tokyo and other Japanese cities.

Founded as a fortified settlement in the 1450s by the name of Edo (literally "estuary"), the name Tokyo (meaning "Capital of the East") emerged in 1868, with the establishment of the Meiji Era in Japan. Between these two dates, in circa 1619, the Edo Castle was completed, but suffered serious damage in the 1657 Meireki Fire. In 1872 another fire consumed the districts of Ginza and Tsukiji, and yet by the turn of the 19th century Tokyo had more than 800,000 inhabitants. In 1923 the Great Kanto Earthquake destroyed more than half of Tokyo's wooden buildings. Succeeding reconstruction was guided by an ambitious plan with 16 middle-class settlements built between 1925 and 1927. Japan joined World War II as German and Italian allies. In 1941, following the Pearl Harbor bombing, Tokyo suffered 70 air-raids before Hiroshima and Nagasaki were annihilated in 1945, forcing the country to surrender. At the end of the war, more than a fourth of Tokyo had been destroyed, and it's population had dropped by four million.

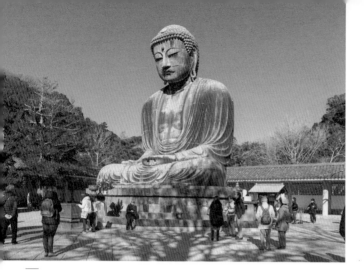

Figure 18.3
The monumental bronze Amida Buddha in Kamakura
Source: Kakidai (see Image Credits for details)

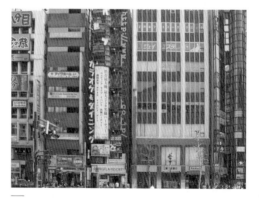

Figure 18.4
Tall, thin buildings in Tokyo resulting from the literal vertical extrusion of small lots
Source: Author

But the 1950s saw not only an overwhelming population increase, but also the beginnings of even greater economic growth. A lot of this rebirth, in the physical sense, happened largely without formal planning. The proposals in the '50s included decentralization at both a regional and city scale through the creation of multiple centers - beginning with Shibuya, Ikebukuro, and Shinjuku; followed by Asakusa, Osaki, and Kameido; and eventually spreading into the reclaimed islands within the Tokyo Bay. The government initially followed this post-war recovery plan focusing on infrastructure and disaster relief, but gradually, deviating from the plan's most ambitious recommendations, left housing and commercial development to local forces.

Public housing entities did build dwellings for the more needy classes, but this was a small part of the 11 million new dwelling units that cropped up between the late '50s and early '70s. Most were single-family ownership homes and modest rental units, all managed by private parties and created by the local construction industry relying on homeowner participation and traditional building practices. By 1960, Tokyo had more than nine million residents, living in an expensive city that had in a desperate drive of rapid reconstruction swallowed up its surrounding countryside. Tokyo's urban evolution is unique in this regard, revealing spasms of urban explosion and destruction, and their replacement with new urban patterns and grids previously unseen. Only Edo Castle remains a visual reference point in this city.

Living with uncertainty and massive change is not new to Japan. Consider, for instance, its traditional choice of timber - a building material vulnerable to the perils of fires and natural disasters. As a result, there is not a single traditional monument in Japan today that has not been rebuilt. The Great Buddha Hall of the Todai-ji Temple in Nara, once the largest wooden building the world, has been rebuilt twice after its destruction by fire. In 1730, when the Great Nishijin Fire destroyed Kyoto's Imperial Palace yet again, the Shogun simply ordered its reconstruction on an even grander scale, only to be burnt again in 1854 and replicated to its current form. The monumental bronze Amida Buddha in Kamakura that sits under the sky was originally sheltered in a temple that was destroyed numerous times.

Even before Buddhism arrived in 538 CE, Japan's early Shinto traditions had maintained that divine *kami* (nature spirits) dwell intermittently in natural elements such a trees and mountains, and through this cyclical possession, bring about a constant flux in the perceived nature of the place. The establishment of Buddhism with its philosophical emphasis on transience and change reinforced this Shinto sensitivity to temporality. The Japanese acknowledgment to changing seasons, rebuilding of their shrines and habitats, their unique attitude toward unpredictable events, must all be understood as the evolution of a deep cultural psychology shaped as much by religion and philosophy as the fragile ecology in which the culture is rooted.

In Japanese cities today, disaster preparedness is at work at all scales. In major cities, each district has an evacuation spot, emergency road, and temporary facilities with hazard maps showing areas of possible major damage and fire. In Tokyo, around 200 locations are registered for temporary emergencies including local parks, public schools, gas stations, and convenience stores. Following the Tohoku Earthquake and tsunami in 2012, the Tokyo Metropolitan Government announced a disaster preparation plan that uses the city's fire hydrants as water stations for shelters in the event of an earthquake or similar disaster. According to the local government's Bureau of Waterworks, roughly 130,000 fire hydrants throughout the city will be able to provide fresh water to as many as 5,000 refugee shelters, serving nearly eight million people. To turn fire hydrants into water stations, necessary supplies like water hoses and standpipes have already been distributed to the city's wards and towns.

In February 2020, the COVID-19 pandemic startled Japan, just like the rest of the world. A passenger aboard a cruise ship docked in the port of Yokohama tested positive for the coronavirus six days after leaving the ship, and by February 11, as many as 1,850 people on board had requested and received prescription medications. By the end of March, 2020, the situation had intensified leading to weekend lockdowns. On April 7, Japan's Prime Minister declared a national emergency, encouraging physical distancing to control the virus spread. And all this came amidst Japan's announcement of postponing the 2020 Olympic Games by a year due to the pandemic, putting greater pressure on its already stressed economy. As we all grapple with the COVID-19 pandemic, it will be worthwhile to see how Japan's long history of coping with crises will shape its receptions to this one. It will be insightful to observe whether Japanese cities will engage with these uncertain times differently from the rest of us.

How would you live in a city that you know will be destroyed from time to time? In Japan, I have witnessed an urban phenomenon where disaster translates into cyclical occurrence, where chaos translates into J. Saramago's definition of an "order to be deciphered," and where density translates into a mechanism for survival. Our perception of cities as permanent entities may well be an exaggeration born out of our inadvertent drive to take numerous socio-economic and environmental aspects for granted. This is exactly what the pandemic has done - whacked us in the head like a Zen master and woken us up to the truism of uncertainty and the constancy of change.

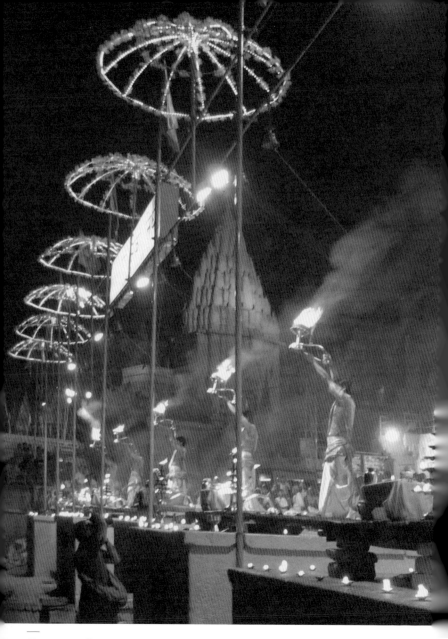

Figure 19.1 **Daily Ganga Puja (ritual worship of Ganga River), Banaras, India.**
Source: Author

19

Learning from Banaras

During this pandemic, I find it particularly meaningful to reflect on the Indian city of Banaras. One of the things this pandemic has done is overturned many aspects of our cities that we take for granted. Who would have thought that we would spend more than a year sitting six feet apart from each other? Or go for months largely confined to our homes? Across continents and nations, the pandemic has expanded our perspective on cities, and Banaras, more than any other city in the world, has in a different way done exactly this for me - challenged my preconceptions of what cities are and ought to be.

All streets in Banaras lead ultimately to the eastern bank of the Ganga River, which is today the sixth-most polluted river in the world, largely due to toxic industrial waste. During India's pandemic lockdown in 2020, with factories closed, and daily worship and cremations stopped, the river was cleaner than it has been in decades. Over the years, numerous deliberations had concluded that cleaning the river would be possible only with consensus from all users and stakeholders - a difficult task considering their varying interests and priorities. The pandemic made possible what none of us could.

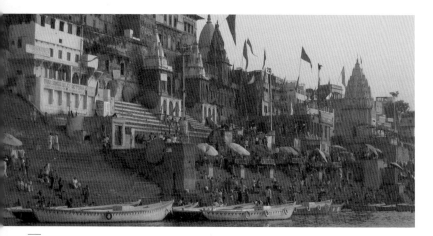

Figure 19.2
Dashashwamedha Ghat, Banaras, India
Source: Author

In Banaras, which is the holiest of the seven sacred Hindu cities in India, the Ganga's eastern bank is a six-kilometer-long sacred confluence of land and water with eighty-four *ghats* (stepped streets with platforms, temples, and shrines) cascading down a concave riverbank. The number eighty-four refers to the cosmic order of 12 zodiacs and the seven atmospheric layers. Each ghat represents 100,000 *yoni* (organic species) described in Hindu mythology, and it is believed that by taking dips in the river at all the ghats, one's soul can get purified in all the 84,000 species that encompass existence. Among the 84 ghats, five are considered to be *panchatirthis* (the most merit-giving): Asi, Dashashvamedha, Manikarnika, Panchaganga, and Adi Keshava.

The ghats are punctuated by innumerable shrines of all sizes and forms making it a gallery of sacred art that is as exotic to a tourist as cognizable to the pious who use it each day. At the Dashash-

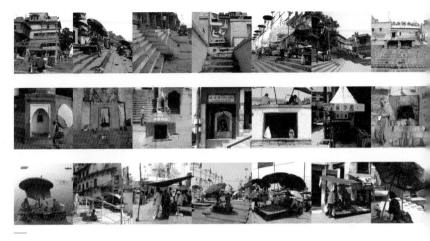

Figure 19.3
**Photographic analysis of the *ghats* as a sacredscape. From top to bottom rows:
Steps, Shrines, and Activities**
Source: Vinayak Bharne & Ashrita Hegde

vamedha Ghat, each morning, devotees come down the steps to the river to bathe and pray. Temple bells awaken the gods, platforms are set up for daily activity, thatched parasols are erected, and wooden desks displayed with myriad sacred fetishes. Within hours the riverbank transforms into a maze of sacred commerce with flower vendors, fortune tellers, and pilgrims. After sundown, the platforms are cleaned and the ghat is transformed into a stage for the river's daily worship. Young monks from proximate temples and monasteries perform a synchronized *aarti* (lamp display) along with chants in a spectacular ritual called the Ganga Puja. This daily worship of the Ganga River was being conducted by a single priest without any public audience during India's 2020 COVID-19 lockdown. That the authorities found a way to keep the ritual going amidst this uncertain time, affirms what sacredness means in this city.

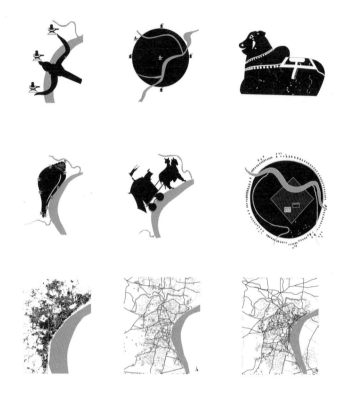

Figure 19.4
Different perceptions of Banaras. Mappings of the city done by pilgrims, priests and artists (top and middle rows) versus those done by surveyors, planners and architects (bottom row)
Source: Vinayak Bharne & Ashrita Hegde

The sacred landscape of Banaras is a much larger spatial system however, manifested in a series of pilgrimage circuits, each marked by a finite number of "stations" embodied in temples and shrines. There are about 108 different pilgrimage circuits, each originally associated with different purposes and deities. Many have lost their identities, but around 52 survive to varying degrees in five sacred territories. Taken together, they contain 468 temples, shrines, and sacred sites, representing the integration of nine planets, 13 months (12 plus one inter-calary), and the four directions.

The Panchakroshi Yatra is the most popular of the pilgrimages, covering a distance of around 88 kilometers. It has a total of 108 sacred sites, the number stemming from the summation of 12 months of the year and the nine planets of Hindu cosmogony (*nava graha*). This journey, believed to provide purification from all types of sins, is divided into five parts and identified with five halting spots where pilgrims can stay overnight in rest houses. Pilgrims visit a total of 72 temples and shrines, representing the integration of nine planets, four cardinal directions, and the two opposite sides of a day - light versus dark.

Most of us visiting Banaras would not understand the symbolic significance of the ghats and circuits. Even if we walked along a pilgrimage path, we would find nothing special about it, because these routes are neither marked nor visually celebrated. In fact, they are interfaced with the mundane city - amidst driving cars, informal shacks, wayside shrines, and ordinary buildings. For visitors, Banaras is an exotic city of temples, spires, and stepped terraces. But for innumerable residents and the pious, it is what Rana P. B. Singh, one of the world's foremost scholars on Banaras today, calls a "faithscape" - that transcends the physical appearance of the city.

This difference is evident in city mappings done by professional surveyors and architects versus pilgrims and local priests. The surveys align Banaras with north pointing to the top. They depict the arc of the Ganga River from the south-west to north-east with the labyrinthine cityscape of tenuous lanes, water bodies and buildings. By contrast, drawings by pilgrims, priests and cultural geographers depict Banaras as a sacred diagram, emphasizing its temples, circuits, and cosmic symbolisms. None of these mappings by themselves tell us the full story. But taken together, they reveal the complex layers that constitute the experience of the city - from the objective and physical to the cognitive and personal.

Banaras reminds us that our cities and its events are understood differently by different users and that their modes of reading are not the same. Our experience of a city stems as much from our personal predilections as the beliefs of others that may or may not influence our own.

In Fall 2013, as if to test this idea, I conducted a semester-long experimental lab in Banaras with 16 graduate students from the University of Southern California with multidisciplinary backgrounds - urban planning, public health, public administration, architecture, psychology, economics, finance, and non-government-organization-management. We reversed the obvious investigation process: the visit to Banaras was not in the early weeks, but the latter part of the semester - intended not as an analytical survey of the urban condition, but a keen verification exercise, testing firsthand the validity of our ideas and concepts contemplated from a distance with citizens and local agents. Relying on videos, readings, and digital conversations with scholars during the semester, we generated plausible urban transformation strategies for the city, knowing well that our ideas were speculative and even naïve.

In the final two weeks, we visited Banaras for 10 days. We set out to test the validity of our proposals with a broad demographic section - from vendors and professors to hermits and municipal authorities. The result was a transformative series of edits, corrections, and new ideas based on field observations, and far more importantly, invaluable local feedback. We presented the difference between our original and new propositions to faculty and local professionals at Banaras Hindu University and then CEPT University. We candidly highlighted the shifting epiphanies and revelations that had dawned on us through the process of transitioning from mere observers of Banaras, to actually engaging with the city first-hand.

We had discovered "many Banarases." There was one that continues to fascinate tourist, scholar, and architect - a physical landscape of steps, temples, and shrines. There was another in the vast cognitive sacred-scape perceived by pilgrims and priests. A third Banaras was the contemporary Indian city gripped with a housing shortage, water crisis, traffic congestion, extreme economic polarization, and social oppression. And the fourth was the domain of the municipality, struggling to administer this bewildering city through conventional planning instruments such as Floor Space Index (FSI,) zoning, and master plans. Our engagement with Banaras had therefore resulted in a complex muddle of ideas - top-down and bottom-up, physical and non-physical, dealing with mobility, land-use, infrastructure, social-reform, religion, and urban growth, and in both the historic and growing city - revealing the complex interrelationships between Banaras's sacred and mundane dimensions.

What we truly learned is that by letting go of our preconceptions about Banaras, we had uncovered pointers to its future that we could never have hoped to find as erudite experts from a distance. By engaging, however imperfectly, with the numerous local voices that knew their city far better than we ever would, we had evolved from being expert outsiders to empathetic collaborators. By changing the vantage point from where we read the city, we had learnt to acknowledge the multiple realities that embodied it, whether they seemed quaint and anachronistic to some, or perfectly ordinary to others. Banaras taught us that there can be many "normals," and there can even be "new normals" - as the COVID-19 pandemic is showing us.

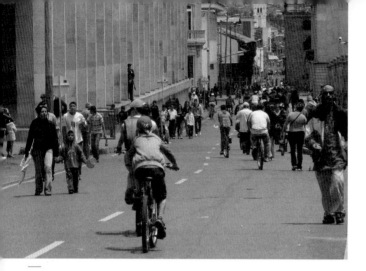

Figure 20.1
Ciclovia in Bogota, Colombia, circa 2009
Source: Nati_fg (see Image Credits for details)

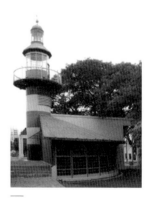

Figure 20.2
Lighthouses of Knowledge project in Curitiba, Brazil
Source: Public Domain

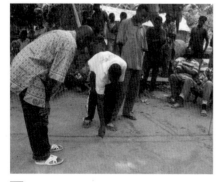

Figure 20.3
A participatory planning session in Central Africa Source: Public Domain

20

The Pawn and the Chess Game

As the pandemic shakes up our economies and real estate markets, architects, urban designers, and city planners are realizing that we are pawns in the chess game of city making. How much power do we really wield when it comes to making the most significant decisions on the future of our cities? Aren't we brought into the picture after important aspects - such as the location and budget of a project - are already established? We work within a framework of constraints and limitations, be it bureaucratic entitlement processes or laborious zoning codes. We have to navigate the agendas of our politicians on the one hand and negotiate the whims of citizens and communities on the other. We are neither rooks nor knights on the chess board of city making, and we are most certainly not the kings and queens.

The pandemic has triggered many important architectural questions related to our dwellings, neighborhoods, and public spaces that we architects and urban designers are far better equipped to discuss and opine on than other disciplines. But putting these ideas into action, finding the financial means to enable them, and garnering support for them is not the same thing. The pandemic has reminded us of our disciplinary limitations and highlighted why collective engagement is superior to a single architectural or planning mind. It has underscored the importance of being open to a constant feedback loop from other disciplines and entities, acknowledging our interdependence, learning from one another, and maturing together through a constant nurturing process.

Isn't it tragic that the architecture and city planning fields - two disciplines that share the same goal of shaping the city - are not inextricably intertwined? There was a time when they were. Why did we segregate ourselves into specialized silos? If architects were engaged in reforming our zoning codes, if planners in turn took interest in the quality of the physical places we build, if civil engineers received training in ecological issues, if landscape architects did not preoccupy themselves exclusively with the open spaces between buildings, and if we all collectively made sure to involve our communities as essential and intrinsic participants in the city making process, our cities would be treading a very different path to their future.

One of the most crucial aspects of our architectural and urbanist engagement is therefore to acknowledge the various other entities that shape our cities - from civic leaders to citizens - and also to realize that ultimately, the city is as much about human agency as larger structures. At the end of the day, cities are created and recreated not in the guise of one person's or one groups' vision, but as a messy muddle of multiple interventions by numerous entities.

"This indeed is practice in the best sense of the term," as Aseem Inam has so astutely noted, "not as a master architect or urbanist, but as one of the many actors who shape the city within a given set of conditions and circumstances. As authors, scholars, and professionals, we practice in all these ways: by instigating questions, by highlighting thematic areas for investigation and discourse, and, finally, by indulging in propositions, whether in staking out positions or creating visions of the future. Practice is ultimately about transformation, even though the vast majority of interventions may fall short." Our efforts may involve the invention of new ideas, rekindling of dormant circumstances, implementation of physical projects, or even discovery of accidental successes. The nature of our practice may be grassroots or utopian. Whatever the case, the central thread running through them all is our willingness to take responsibility for the city.

Today, numerous forms of grass-roots urbanism, also termed as "bottom-up urbanism," "do-it-yourself (DIY) urbanism," "guerilla urbanism," "tactical urbanism," etc., are being seen as essential sparks of brilliance and hope for our urban future. These efforts, most often led by activists and non-government organizations, are seeing uncanny success on issues, and in places where formal urbanist practice has failed to make any relevant impact. Many such practices and initiatives continue to remain below the radar and need to be highlighted and brought into mainstream dialogues on the future of our cities.

In cities heavily controlled by local or national authorities, marginalized communities have long sought to subvert top-down control by providing alternate solutions or defying conventional and permitted practices, often as a reaction to dismal administrative performance. From self-help strategies, micro-finance tactics, and awareness-based interventions, to temporary farmers markets and community gardens, such insurgent efforts challenge our normative ideas of what city making is. They diffuse multiple professions and disciplines toward a common advocacy for a better urban future. They transcend political affiliation making them unsettling to many authorities, and this is where their true power lies.

India, for instance, has more than three-million non-government-organizations, more than any other country in the world, and there is no question that the success of many of these entities with some of the most gripping urban issues - poverty, the informal economy, social injustice, etc. - are things we architecture and planning professionals should constantly learn from.

But this said, to what degree do such grass-roots efforts offer solutions to the myriad other pressing problems plaguing our cities? What about rampant sprawl and rapacious capitalism? Or the looming water crisis? Or the erasure of rural and agrarian landscapes? Or the debacle of single-use zoning and Floor Area Ratio regulations? These issues are equally pressing, for they are destroying the long-term viability of cities across the world by the minute.

They cannot be resolved by modest bottom-up tactics, but by ambitious and visionary long-term planning, where every investment - be it in transit, real-estate, infrastructure, regulation - is synergized as an interdependent socio-economic opportunity. They can only be resolved by clear alternatives that seek to retool the same petrified processes that have perpetrated the current urban condition. In cities with the dire need for such large-scale transformation - not just small-scale interventions - grassroots urbanism offers only short-term sporadic sparks, instead of much-needed waves of reform and long-term change. Bottom-up tactics are necessary band-aids for short-term relief, but they are not the antidote to long-term urban health - be it in Mumbai or Los Angeles.

If, as Michel de Certeau has noted, "tactics" are employed by citizens to negotiate daily life in the city, and "strategies" in turn emanate from the state and corporation in the form of government regulation, what we need are mechanisms that will help transition tactics toward strategy. The city of Bogota, for instance - thanks to a progressive mayor - has undergone major reforms in infrastructure and public transit. The planning department prioritized the improvement of bike lanes, buses, and light rail over vehicular roads. It also simultaneously initiated the first Ciclovia, a weekly event in which over 70 miles of city streets are closed to traffic and opened to walking, biking, recreating, and talking with neighbors and strangers - a concept now picking up in several cities across the world.

Another example is the city of Curitiba's "Farois de Saber" (Light-houses of Knowledge) project, wherein 50 brightly colored, light-house-shaped towers were built throughout the city's low-income neighborhoods. They are free educational centers that include libraries, internet access, and other cultural resources for citizens of all ages, diversifying access to knowledge, and expanding formal education. The most important thing is that these ideas and initia-tives have happened without the necessity of guerilla tactics. These initiatives are exemplary, because they emerge from governments, for communities, with intimate collaboration from conception to implementation and follow through.

We need bottom-up practices and their sparks of brilliance. But we also need simultaneous waves - not sparks - of long-term reform, that will enable catalytic, incremental, systematic, and large-scale change beyond isolated interventions, not for a day or a week, but for decades and beyond. The task for us architects and planners is to facilitate these connections and get citizens and activist groups to understand the virtues of collaborative planning and progressive change. This is indeed what participatory practice is all about. It is an inclusive proposition, with top-down, bottom-up and networked efforts all collaborating toward better cities. Our cities deserve this kind of expansive, multi-dimensional engagement.

The sooner we architects and planners realize our place as pawns in a larger chess game of city making, the better. A pawn on a chess-board can do many things a rook or king cannot. But if a pawn behaved like a knight or rook, all hell would break loose. Now if the same pawn worked strategically with the rooks, bishops, and other pawns, they could collectively enable a wonderful checkmate. If the COVID-19 pandemic teaches architects and planners anything, it is to transform the processes through which our cities are being shaped. We must facilitate strategic multi-disciplinary engagement in the best sense of the term. We must, *collaboratively,* deliberate and propose, succeed or fall short, but either way, learn, get up, and try again, in a never-ending commitment to transform our cities.

Image Credits

Every attempt has been made to appropriately acknowledge image sources. Should there be any errors or omissions, the author and publisher would be pleased to insert the appropriate acknowledgement in any subsequent edition of the book.

Figure 1.1 - Plan of London. Source: Public Domain (https://en.wikipedia.org/wiki/Public_domain)

Figure 1.2 - Plan of Philadelphia. Source: Public Domain (https://en.wikipedia.org/wiki/Public_domain)

Figure 2.1 - La Rambla. Source: Nikos Roussos; licensed under the Creative Commons Attribution-Share Alike 2.0 Generic (https://creativecommons.org/licenses/by-sa/2.0/deed.en)

Figure 2.2 - Korowai tree house. Source: Vinayak Bharne & Nicolle Cotes Chong

Figure 2.3 - Amazon rainforest, Brazil. Source: Andre Deak; licensed under the Creative Commons Attribution 2.0 Generic license (https://creativecommons.org/licenses/by/2.0/deed.en)

Figure 2.4 - Forest depletion. Source: Dikshajhingan; licensed under the Creative Commons Attribution-Share Alike 4.0 International license (https://creativecommons.org/licenses/by-sa/4.0/deed.en)

Figure 3.1 - Turtles. Source: Iryanaraya; licensed under the Creative Commons Attribution-Share Alike 4.0 International license (https://creativecommons.org/licenses/by-sa/4.0/deed.en)

Figure 3.2 - Wildlife overpass. Source: WikiPedant; licensed under the Creative Commons Attribution-Share Alike 4.0 International license (https://creativecommons.org/licenses/by-sa/4.0/deed.en)

Figure 4.1 – Street sweeper. Source: Vinayak Bharne

Figure 4.2 - The Metrocable system. Source: Jorge Láscar; licensed under the Creative Commons Attribution 2.0 Generic license (https://creativecommons.org/licenses/by/2.0/deed.en)

Figure 4.3 - Bus Rapid Transit system. Source: Mario Roberto Duran Ortiz; licensed under the Creative Commons Attribution-Share Alike 3.0 Unported license (https://creativecommons.org/licenses/by-sa/3.0/deed.en)

Figure 4.4 - Escalator in Medellin. Source: Juan Gómez; licensed under the Creative Commons Attribution 2.0 Generic license (https://creativecommons.org/licenses/by/2.0/deed.en)

Figure 5.1/5.2/5.3/5.4 - Source: Vinayak Bharne

Figure 6.1 - Narakasur. Source: Siddha Sardessai

Figure 6.2 - Ganesh Festival parade. Source: Ninadism; licensed under the Creative Commons Attribution 2.0 Generic license (https://creativecommons.org/licenses/by/2.0/deed.en)

Figure 6.3 - Gion Matsuri. Source: Noboru Asano

Figure 7.1 - Town Hall, Stockholm. Source: W. Bulach; This is a partial view of an original photo licensed under the Creative Commons Attribution-Share Alike 4.0 International license (https://creativecommons.org/licenses/by-sa/4.0/deed.en). For original photo see https://commons.wikimedia.org/wiki/File:00_5252_Stockholm_City_Hall,_Centralbron.jpg

Figure 8.1 - Panaji Church Square. Source: Vinayak Bharne

Figure 8.2 - Plaza Mayor. Source: Sebastian Dubiel; licensed under the Creative Commons Attribution-Share Alike 3.0 Germany license (https://creativecommons.org/licenses/by-sa/3.0/de/deed.en)

Figure 8.3 - Naqsh-e Jahan Square. Source: Arosha-photo(Reza Sobhani); This file is licensed under the Creative Commons Attribution-Share Alike 4.0 International (https://creativecommons.org/licenses/by-sa/4.0/deed.en) license)

Figure 8.4 - Regent Street. Source: Jon Curnow; This file is licensed under the Creative Commons Attribution 2.0 Generic license (https://creativecommons.org/licenses/by/2.0/deed.en)

Figure 8.5 - Plan of Kyoto. Source: Vinayak Bharne

Figure 8.6 - Registan Square. Source: LBM1948; This file is licensed under the Creative Commons Attribution-Share Alike 4.0 International license (https://creativecommons.org/licenses/by-sa/4.0/deed.en)

Figure 9.1 - Lower Manhattan. Source: Sam Valadi; This file is licensed under the Creative Commons Attribution 2.0 Generic license (https://creativecommons.org/licenses/by/2.0/deed.en)

Figure 9.2 - Plan Voisin. Source: SiefkinDR; This file is licensed under the Creative Commons Attribution-Share Alike 4.0 International license (https://creativecommons.org/licenses/by-sa/4.0/deed.en)

Figure 10.1/10.2 - Source: Vinayak Bharne

Figure 10.3 - Urban Agriculture, Cuba. Source: Arnoud Joris Maaswinkel; This file is licensed under the Creative Commons Attribution-Share Alike 4.0 International license (https://creativecommons.org/licenses/by-sa/4.0/deed.en)

Figure 11.1 - Ginza. Source: Vinayak Bharne

Figure 11.2 - Belfast, Maine. Source: Bruce C. Cooper; Centpacrr at en.wikipedia (https://en.wikipedia.org). This file is licensed under the Creative Commons Attribution-Share Alike 3.0 Unported license (https://creativecommons.org/licenses/by-sa/3.0/deed.en)

Figure 11.3 - Santa Fe, Mexico. Source: Serge Saint (https://www.flickr.com/photos/sergiosf/). This file is licensed under the Creative Commons Attribution 2.0 Generic license (https://creativecommons.org/licenses/by/2.0/deed.en)

Figure 11.4 - Source: Vinayak Bharne

Figure 12.1 - Floating market. Source: Muhammad Haris. This file is licensed under the Creative Commons Attribution-Share Alike 4.0 International license (https://creativecommons.org/licenses/by-sa/4.0/deed.en). This is a partial version of the original. For original image, see https://commons.wikimedia.org/w/index.php?title=File:Jukung_Pasar_Terapung.jpg&oldid=557495984

Figure 12.2 - Tusha Hiti. Source: Bijaya2043; This file is licensed under the Creative Commons Attribution-Share Alike 4.0 International license (https://creativecommons.org/licenses/by-sa/4.0/deed.en).

Figure 12.3 - Chand Baori. Source: Gryffindor. This file is made available under the Creative Commons CC0 1.0 Universal Public Domain Dedication (https://creativecommons.org/publicdomain/zero/1.0/deed.en).

Figure 12.4 - Qanats in Yazd, Iran. Source: Vinayak Bharne & Biayna Bogosian

Figure 13.1 - India Gate. Source: Gughanbose; This file is licensed under the Creative Commons Attribution 3.0 Unported license (https://creativecommons.org/licenses/by/3.0/deed.en)

Figure 13.2 - Jantar Mantar. Source: Abhijit Jawanjal; This file is licensed under the Creative Commons Attribution 3.0 Unported license (https://creativecommons.org/licenses/by/3.0/deed.en)

Figure 13.3 - Open Hand. Photo: Vinayak Bharne; Copyright 2010 Artists Rights Society (ARCS), New York/ADAGP, Paris/F.L.C.

Figure 14.1 - Plan of Rome. Source: Public Domain; This file has been identified as being free of known restrictions under copyright law, including all related and neighboring rights. (https://creativecommons.org/publicdomain/mark/1.0/deed.en)

Figure 14.2 - Qingming Shanghe Tu. Source: Immanuel Giel; Public Domain; This file has been identified as being free of known restrictions under copyright law, including all related and neighboring rights. (https://creativecommons.org/publicdomain/mark/1.0/deed.en)

Figure 14.3 - Japanese Silk Screen. Source: Public Domain; This file has been identified as being free of known restrictions under copyright law, including all related and neighboring rights. (https://creative-commons.org/publicdomain/mark/1.0/deed.en)

Figure 14.4 - Regent Street. Source: Simeon87; This file is licensed under the Creative Commons Attribution-Share Alike 4.0 International license (https://creativecommons.org/licenses/by-sa/4.0/deed.en). This is a partial version of the original. For original image, see https://commons.wikimedia.org/wiki/File:Regent_Street_Christmas_2017_Decorations.jpg

Figure 14.5 - Japanese paper lantern. Source: Vinayak Bharne

Figure 14.6 - Santa Marta favela. Source: André Sampaio; This file is licensed under the Creative Commons Attribution 3.0 Unported license (https://creativecommons.org/licenses/by/3.0/deed.en)

Figure 14.7 - "Coronavirus" art installation. Source: Vinayak Bharne

Figure 15.1 - The Pont du Gard. Source: Roberto Ferrari; This file is licensed under the Creative Commons Attribution-Share Alike 2.0 Generic license (https://creativecommons.org/licenses/by-sa/2.0/deed.en).

Figure 15.2 - Shinkansen bullet train. Source: Tansaisuketti; This file is licensed under the Creative Commons Attribution 3.0 Unported license (https://creativecommons.org/licenses/by/3.0/deed.en).

Figure 16.1 - Yoyogi Stadium. Source: Vinayak Bharne

Figure 16.2 – Chandigarh. Photo: Vinayak Bharne; Copyright 2010 Artists Rights Society (ARCS), New York/ADAGP, Paris/F.L.C.

Figure 16.3 - Taj Mahal. Source: Vinayak Bharne

Figure 17.1 - Map of Shanghai. Source: Public Domain (https://en.wikipedia.org/wiki/Public_domain)

Figure 17.2 – Puxi. Source: Public Domain (https://en.wikipedia.org/wiki/Public_domain)

Figure 17.3 – Pudong. Source: This file is made available under the Creative Commons CC0 1.0 Universal Public Domain Dedication (https://creativecommons.org/publicdomain/zero/1.0/deed.en).

Figure 17.4/17.5/17.6 - Source: Vinayak Bharne

Figure 18.1 - Cityscape of Tokyo. Source: Michael Greenhalgh (courtesy of ArtServe)

Figure 18.2 - Evolution of Tokyo. Source: Vinayak Bharne

Figure 18.3 - Amida Buddha. Source: Kakidai; This file is licensed under the Creative Commons Attribution-Share Alike 4.0 International license (https://creativecommons.org/licenses/by-sa/4.0/deed.en)

Figure 18.4/19.1/19.2 - Source: Vinayak Bharne

Figure 19.3/19.4 - Source: Vinayak Bharne & Ashrita Hegde

Figure 20.1 - Ciclovia. Source: Nati_fg; This file is licensed under the Creative Commons Attribution 2.0 Generic license (https://creativecommons.org/licenses/ by/2.0/deed.en)

Figure 20.2 – Lighthouses of Knowledge. Source: Public Domain (https://en.wikipedia.org/wiki/Public_domain)

Figure 20.3 - Participatory planning. Source: Public Domain

References

1. Our Health and the City

For more on the history and planning of Philadelphia, see Mann Emily, "Story of cities #7: Philadelphia grid marks birth of America's urban dream," in *The Guardian,* March 22, 2016; https://www.theguardian.com/cities/2016/mar/22/story-of-cities-7-philadelphia-grid-pennsylvania-william-penn-america-urban-dream, accessed in July 2021

For more on the history of Central Park, New York, see Blackmar Elizabeth and Rosenzweig Roy, *The Park and the People: A History of Central Park,* Cornell University Press, 1992

For more on health crisis in the history of the United States, see Carr Sara Jensen's forthcoming book, *The Topography of Wellness: How Health and Disease Shaped the American Urban Landscape, 1840–Present,* University of Virginia Press, 2021. It will offer a chronological narrative of how six epidemics transformed the American urban landscape.

For more on the thoughts and ideas of Patrick Geddes, see Tyrwhitt Jaqueline (editor), *Patrick Geddes in India,* Lund Humphries, London 1947, pg 66 -83

2. The Forest and the City

For more on the deforestation and infectious diseases, see Bloomfield, L.S.P., McIntosh, T.L. & Lambin, E.F. "Habitat fragmentation, livelihood behaviors, and contact between people and nonhuman primates in Africa." *Landscape Ecology,* 35, 985–1000 (2020). https://doi.org/10.1007/s10980-020-00995-w

For more on the "empty forest" phenomenon, see Kent H. Redford; "The Empty Forest", *BioScience,* Volume 42, Issue 6, June 1992, Pages 412–422

For more on the impact of the pandemic on climate change, see Piers M. Forster, Harriet I. Forster, Mat J. Evans, Matthew J. Gidden, Chris D. Jones, Christoph A. Keller, Robin D. Lamboll, Corinne Le Quéré, Joeri Rogelj, Deborah Rosen, Carl-Friedrich Schleussner, Thomas B. Richardson, Christopher J. Smith & Steven T. Turnock, "Current and future global climate impacts resulting from COVID-19." *Nature Climate Change* 10, 913–919 (2020). https://doi.org/10.1038/s41558-020-0883-0

3. The Wild City

For more on wildlife conservation, see Clevenger Anthony P. and Waltho Nigel, "Factors Influencing the Effectiveness of Wildlife Underpasses in Banff National Park, Alberta, Canada"; *Conservation Biology,* Vol. 14, No. 1 (Feb., 2000), pp. 47-56

For more on the concept of "rewilding," see Soulè Michael and Noss Reed, "Rewilding and Biodiversity: Complimentary Goals for Continental Conservation," *Wild Earth,* Fall 1998, Vol. 8. No. 3, pp. 2-11

For more on Multispecies Urbanism, see Solomon Debra, "Multispecies Urbanism: Introduction," in *Openresearch.Amsterdam;* https://openresearch.amsterdam/en/page/56483/multispecies-urbanism-introduction, accessed in June 2021

4. The Unfair City

For more on Bogota, Colombia's transit systems, see https://www.transmilenio.gov.co/publicaciones/noticias/?tema=12; accessed July 2021

For more on Curitiba's Bus Rapid Transit system, see "How Curitiba's BRT stations sparked a transport revolution," in *The Guardian,* May 26, 2015; https://www.theguardian.com/cities/2015/may/26/curitiba-brazil-brt-transport-revolution-history-cities-50-buildings; accessed July 2021

For more on social housing in the Netherlands, see Khandekar Siddharth, "Dutch Social Housing Today," Chapter 20, pg. 121-123 in Bharne Vinayak & Khandekar Shyam (editors), *Affordable Housing, Inclusive Cities,* My Liveable City & ORO Editions, 2019.

5. The Informal City

For more on vendors and the pandemic, see "For World's Street Vendors, Life May Never be the Same after COVID-19;" https://www.wiego.org/blog/worlds-street-vendors-life-may-never-be-same-after-covid-19; accessed July 2021

For more on wayside shrines, see Bharne Vinayak, "Anointed Cities: The Incremental Urbanism of Hindu India," Chapter 1, pg. 17-26 in Bharne Vinayak (editor), *The Emerging Asian City: Concomitant Urbanities & Urbanisms,* Routledge, London 2013.

For more on informal urbanism in the context of south Asia, see Perera Nihal, *People's Spaces: Coping, Familiarizing, Creating,* Routledge; London, 1st edition October 29, 2015

For more on the idea of the "kinetic city," see Mehrotra Rahul, "The Static & The Kinetic," in *Urban Age, LSE Cities,* October 2013; (https://urbanage.lsecities.net/essays/the-static-and-the-kinetic) accessed June 2021

6. The Privilege of Community

For an informative video of the organization, preparation and details of the Gion Maturi festival, see "Gion Matsuri: The Hokaboko Float's Journey," *Discover Kyoto,* February 2015; https://www.youtube.com/watch?v=yDmKBun19nA, accessed in July 2021

For a video of the Ganesh festivities in the city of Mumbai, India, see "Mumbai's Biggest cultural event," *Hemant Pictures,* August 2019; (https://www.youtube.com/watch?v=z5qitJerfbM) accessed in July 2021

7. Governance Matters

For more on the pandemic as a socio-political challenge in Africa, see Chinedu Josephine Onyishi, Adaeze UP Ejike-Alieji, Chukwuedozie Kelechukwu Ajaero, Casmir Chukwuka Mbaegbu, Christian Chukwuebuka Ezeibe, Victor Udemezue Onyebueke, Peter Oluchukwu Mbah, Thaddeus Chidi Nzeadibe; "COVID-19 Pandemic and Informal Urban Governance in Africa: A Political Economy Perspective," first published in *Journal of Asian and African Studies,* Sage Journals, September 30, 2020; https://doi.org/10.1177/0021909620960163 accessed January, 2021

For more on community support during the pandemic in South Asia, see "COVID-19 Support in South Asia: Organizations and Citizen Initiatives," published by the *Henry M. Jackson School of International Studies, South Asia Center,* University of Washington, April 3, 2020; https://jsis.washington.edu/southasia/news/covid-19-support-in-south-asia/ accessed in April 2020

8. Paradigms of Open Space

For more on Compliance Protocols for POPS during the pandemic, see "DCP Compliance Protocol," New York City Department of Planning, https://www1.nyc.gov/site/planning/about/dcp-compliance-protocol.page, accessed July 2021

9. The High-rise City

For more on the densest cities in the world, see "Population Density By City," published by *World Population Review;* https://worldpopulationreview.com/world-city-rankings/population-density-by-city accessed in March 2021

For more on COVID-19 and High-rise buildings, see Morley David, "COVID in the City: High-rise Building, Elevator Lifts & Fallen Symbols," in *Inter-Asia Cultural Studies,* Volume 21, 2020; Issue 4, pg 614-621. Published online by Taylor & Francis Online on December 18, 2020 (https://www.tandfonline.com/doi/full/10.1080/14649373.2020.1831810), accessed July 2021.

10. Shaping the Polycentric City

For more on the efficacy of the Neighborhood Unit concept beyond the West, see Nahyang Byun, Youngjun Choi & Jaepil Choi, "The Neighborhood Unit: Effective or Obsolete?, *Journal of Asian Architecture and Building Engineering,* 13:3, 617-624, 2014; https://doi.org/10.3130/jaabe.13.617, accessed July 2021

For more on zoning in Japan, see Gray Nolan, "Why Is Japanese Zoning More Liberal Than US Zoning?", published in *Market Urbanism,* March 2019; https://marketurbanism.com/2019/03/19/why-is-japanese-zoning-more-liberal-than-us-zoning/ accessed June 2021

For more on urban farming in Cuba, see Clouse Carey, "Cuba's Urban Farming Revolution: How to Create Self-Sufficient Cities," in *Architectural Review,* March 17, 2014

11. Rethinking Retail

For more on Amazon's efforts during the pandemic, see "Amazon has hired 175,000 additional people" written by Amazon staff, June 2020; https://blog.aboutamazon.com/company-news/amazon-hiring-for-additional-75-000-jobs accessed in July 2020

For more on the evolution of retail urbanism in Los Angeles, see Bharne Vinayak, "Designing the Urban Block: Best Practices in Los Angeles," *Practicing Planner* - Fall 2011 - Vol. 9, No. 3, American Planning Association, 2011

For more on the evolution of mega-block retail in Los Angeles, see Longstreth Richard, *City Center to Regional Mall: Architecture, the Automobile and Retailing in Los Angeles, 1920-1950;* The MIT Press; Reprint edition (June 5, 1998)

For more on mall transformations in the United States, see Steuteville Robert, "Malls to Mixed-use Centers and other Opportunities," *Public Square,* Congress for the New Urbanism, October 2019; https://www.cnu.org/publicsquare/2019/10/08/malls-mixed-use-centers-and-other-opportunities, accessed June 2020

For more on retail during and beyond the pandemic, see Evans Michelle, "7 Predictions For How COVID-19 will change Retail in the Future," in *Forbes,* May 2020; https://www.forbes.com/sites/michelleevans1/2020/05/19/7-predictions-for-how-covid-19-will-change-retail-in-the-future/#46fd18945be3, accessed in September 2020

12. Saving Vernacular Urbanisms

For more in water scarcity during the pandemic, see Boretti A. "COVID-19 pandemic as a further driver of water scarcity in Africa" published online ahead of print, *GeoJournal*, 2020, 1-28. doi:10.1007/s10708-020-10280-7, 2020 Aug 25; https://www.ncbi.nlm.nih.gov/pmc/articles/PMC7445842/, accessed in July 2020

For more on the Asia's vernacular water systems, see Bharne Vinayak, "Conserving Asia's Vernacular Water Urbanisms," Chapter 3, pg. 67-79, published in Silva Kapila (editor), *The Routledge Handbook on Historic Urban Landscapes in the Asia-Pacific,* Routledge, London, 2020

13. Narratives of Protest

For more on Shinjuku Concerts, see Andrews Williams, *Dissenting Japan: A History of Japanese Radicalism and Counterculture from 1945 to Fukushima,* Oxford University Press, Aug 15, 2016

For more on the history of Ramlila Maidan, see Nath Dipanita, "Explained: Why the 200-year Ramnagar ki Ramlila has an important place in India's art history," in *The Indian Express,* October 23, 2020; https://indianexpress.com/article/explained/explained-why-the-200-year-ramnagar-ki-ramlila-has-an-important-place-in-indias-art-history-6839744/, accessed in December 2020

For more on New Delhi's air pollution, see Thomas Vinod and Tiwari Chitranjali, "Delhi, the world's most air polluted capital fights back," in *Brookings,* November 25, 2020; https://www.brookings.edu/blog/future-development/2020/11/25/delhi-the-worlds-most-air-polluted-capital-fights-back/, accessed in December 2020

14. The Arts and the City

For more on street art during the pandemic, see Billock Jennifer, "How street artists around the world are reacting to life with COVID-19," published in *Smithsonian Magazine,* April 23, 2020; https://www.smithsonianmag.com/travel/how-street-artists-around-world-are-reacting-to-life-with-covid-19-180974712/, accessed in June 2020

For more on the City of Boulder's COVID-19 art programs, see "COVID-19 Work Projects," City of Boulder Office of Arts and Culture, https://boulderarts.org/public-art/creative-neighborhoods/covid-19-work-projects/, accessed July 2021

15. Technology and the City

For more on digital technology and the pandemic, see Ting, D.S.W., Carin, L., Dzau, V. et al. "Digital technology and COVID-19," in *Nature Medicine,* 26, 459–461, 2020; https://doi.org/10.1038/s41591-020-0824-5, accessed in July 2021

For more on Worldometer, see https://www.worldometers.info/coronavirus/, accessed in July 2021

For the report of the National Statistical Office of the Government of India, 2017-2018, see http://mospi.nic.in/sites/default/files/publication_reports/KI_Education_75th_Final.pdf, accessed in July 2021

For more on online education in India during the pandemic, see Kundu Protiva, "Indian education can't go online – only 8% of homes with young members have computer with net link," in *Scroll.in,* May 2020; https://scroll.in/article/960939/indian-education-cant-go-online-only-8-of-homes-with-school-children-have-computer-with-net-link, accessed in August 2021

For more on the effectiveness of mobile phones in Africa, see Edelstein David, "Making mobile phones work for the poor," in *BBC Future;* https://www.bbc.com/future/article/20121005-making-mobiles-work-for-the-poor, accessed in July 2021

For more on Loon LLC and its record flight, see Candido Salvatore, "312 Days in the Stratosphere," October 2020; https://medium.com/loon-for-all/312-days-in-the-stratosphere-5c50bd233ec5, accessed in June 2021

16. The Edited City

For more on Chandigarh, see Bharne Vinayak, Le Corbusier's Ruin: The Changing Face of Chandigarh's Capitol, *Journal of Architectural Education,* Volume 62, Issue 2, pg. 99 – 112, March 2011

For more on Taj Mahal, see Bharne Vinayak, "The paradise between two worlds: Rereading Taj Mahal and its environs," Chapter 3, pg. 36-45 in Bharne Vinayak (editor), *The Emerging Asian City: Concomitant Urbanities & Urbanisms,* Routledge, London 2013.

17. A View from the Shanghai Bund

For more on the North Bund development, see Yang Jian, "North Bund to become city's next Lujiazui," published in *Shine,* July 1, 2020; https://www.shine.cn/news/metro/2007011383/, accessed in July 2021

For more on the Bund's historic buildings and conservation, see Chang Qing, "A Chinese Approach to Urban Heritage Conservation and Inheritance: Focus on the Contemporary Changes of Shanghai's Historic Spaces," published in Built Heritage 2017 / 3

For more on citywide conservation efforts in Shanghai, see "Shanghai: Lessons in Urban Regeneration and Heritage Conservation," Lecture transcript, Center for Liveable Cities, Singapore, 21 April, 2018; (https://www.clc.gov.sg/docs/default-source/lecture-transcripts/clc-lecture-transcript-20180421-shanghai-lessons-in-urban-regeneration-and-heritage-conservation.pdf

18. Embracing Uncertainty

For more on the evolution of Tokyo, see Bharne Vinayak, *Zen Spaces & Neon Places: Reflections on Japanese Architecture and Urbanism,* Chapter 11, "Rereading Tokyo," pg. 219-245, AR+D Publishing, San Francisco, 2014

19. Learning from Banaras

For more on the cultural complexities of Banaras, see Singh, Rana P.B., *Banaras: Making of India's Heritage City (Planet Earth & Cultural Understanding),* Cambridge Scholars Publishing, London, new edition, October 1, 2009

For more on Panchakroshi Yatra pilgrimage, see Singh, Rana P.B., *Towards the Pilgrimage Archetype: Panchakroshi Yatra of Banaras,* revised-expanded edition, 2016, Pilgrimage and Cosmology Series- 3. Indica Books, Varanasi

20. The Pawn and the Chess Game

For more on urban practice, see Inam Aseem, "Beyond Practice: Urbanism as Creative Political Act", in *Designing Urban Transformation,* first edition, Routledge, London, 2014

For more on the Farois de Sabre project, see https://educacao.curitiba.pr.gov.br/conteudo/farois-do-saber-e-bibliotecas/3814, published by Curitiba Municipal Secretariat of Education, accessed July 2021

For more on the thoughts of Michel de Certeau, see de Certeau Michel, *The Practice of Everyday Life,* University of California Press, Berkeley and Los Angeles, 1988

Index

ORO Editions
Publishers of Architecture, Art, and Design
Gordon Goff: Publisher

www.oroeditions.com
info@oroeditions.com

Published by ORO Editions

Author and Cover Image: Vinayak Bharne
Book and Cover Design: Apurva Ravi
Managing Editor: Jake Anderson

10 9 8 7 6 5 4 3 2 1 First Edition

ISBN: 978-1-954081-07-9

Color Separations and Printing: ORO Group Ltd.
Printed in China.

ORO Editions makes a continuous effort to minimize the overall carbon footprint of its publications. As part of this goal, ORO Editions, in association with Global ReLeaf, arranges to plant trees to replace those used in the manufacturing of the paper produced for its books. Global ReLeaf is an international campaign run by American Forests, one of the world's oldest nonprofit conservation organizations. Global ReLeaf is American Forests' education and action program that helps individuals, organizations, agencies, and corporations improve the local and global environment by planting and caring for trees.